Encyclopedia of Glaucoma: Clinical Approaches

Volume IV

Encyclopedia of Glaucoma: Clinical Approaches Volume IV

Edited by **Abigail Gipe**

FOSTER
ACADEMICS

New Jersey

Published by Foster Academics,
61 Van Reypen Street,
Jersey City, NJ 07306, USA
www.fosteracademics.com

Encyclopedia of Glaucoma: Clinical Approaches
Volume IV
Edited by Abigail Gipe

International Standard Book Number: 978-1-63242-151-7 (Hardback)

Printed in the United States of America.

Contents

Permissions

List of Contributors

Preface

Every book is a source of knowledge and this one is no exception. The idea that led to the conceptualization of this book was the fact that the world is advancing rapidly; which makes it crucial to document the progress in every field. I am aware that a lot of data is already available, yet, there is a lot more to learn. Hence, I accepted the responsibility of editing this book and contributing my knowledge to the community.

Glaucoma is a specialty in ophthalmology that consists of a group of diseases that affect the optic disc and visual fields and is often followed by elevated intraocular pressure. This book is summarised with new topics in glaucoma that have not been covered earlier. It is a well examined and balanced work inclusive of clinical aspects. This book is dedicated to glaucoma experts, general ophthalmologists, amateurs and researchers to increase their knowledge and understand these complex diseases to encourage further investigation for the benefit of the entire humanity.

While editing this book, I had multiple visions for it. Then I finally narrowed down to make every chapter a sole standing text explaining a particular topic, so that they can be used independently. However, the umbrella subject sinews them into a common theme. This makes the book a unique platform of knowledge.

I would like to give the major credit of this book to the experts from every corner of the world, who took the time to share their expertise with us. Also, I owe the completion of this book to the never-ending support of my family, who supported me throughout the project.

Editor

Clinical Aspects

Uveitic Glaucoma

Shimon Rumelt

Additional information is available at the end of the chapter

1. Introduction

Uveitis is the third leading cause of preventable blindness worldwide although its incidence is relatively infrequent. Over 2 million people worldwide may be affected by uveitis. Its prevalence in the States is estimated as 15 per 100,000 and worldwide as 38-730 per 100,000. [1], [2] Females have a higher prevalence and the prevalence in both genders increases with increasing age. [3]

Uveitis may be accompanied by normal, low or high intraocular pressure (IOP). If the IOP is higher than 21mmHg, it is defined as glaucoma and as all the secondary glaucomas, the optic disc and the visual field may be normal. This is in contrast to primary glaucomas, where the high IOP should be accompanied by either abnormal optic disc or visual field or both.

Uveitic glaucoma refers to glaucoma that develops in uveitic patients. The glaucoma in these cases is secondary to or concurrent with uveitis. This is a narrow definition of uveitis and glaucoma even if since it does not include cases of uveitis that develop in glaucoma patients. Uveitic glaucoma is composed of different ocular diseases of different causes and mechanisms. Between 10% and 20% of the uveitis patients develop glaucoma. [4]-[6] The development of glaucoma is more common in chronic than in acute uveitis glaucoma and may reach 46%. [7] There is no predilection to race or gender.

Any uveitis may be accompanied by glaucoma. Nevertheless, in glaucomatocyclitic crisis or Posner Schlossman disease, both intraocular inflammation and high IOP always concur while in others such as Fuchs' heterochromic iridocyclitis they appear in high association or with lesser association.

2. Pathogenesis of uveitic glaucoma

Imbalance between aqueous humour secretion and clearance due to the intraocular inflammation may result in change in IOP. The IOP is often reduced because of hyopsecretion in conjunction with increased uveoscleral outflow. However, the IOP may be also increased due to increase in outflow resistance.

Several mechanisms are involved in the pathogenesis of glaucoma and this group of diseases may be divided to open and closed angle. Open angle is the largest group. In open angle glaucoma, increased outflow resistance is caused by obstruction of the trabecular meshwork by inflammatory cells, plasma proteins, fibrin and/ or debris. All of these are released from the blood vessels due to loss of aqueous-blood barrier and accumulate in the anterior chamber and the angle. Another mechanism is dysfunction of the trabeculocytes caused by toxicity of blood borne-products. This eventually may result in loss of trabeculocytes and scarring. Increased IOP may be caused by cytokines and prostaglandins. A role for the complement component C1qs has been implicated. [8] This component is part of the complement system, which is activated in uveitis. Rho kinases that are released in uveitis may also result in increased IOP. [9], [10]

Corticosteroid-induced glaucoma is another mechanism for open angle glaucoma. It may occur in up to one third of the patients but with impairment of the conventional outflow facility in uveitic patients, it may increase even to 70%. [11] Corticosteroids are being routinely used for uveitis and they can cause this type of open angle glaucoma in any form although it is more common with topical installation. The development of glaucoma depends on the subject susceptibility (corticosteroid responder), dose, duration, type of medication and route of administration. The glaucoma may develop at any time after the initiation of treatment, but usually within 6 weeks. The glaucoma develops due to multiple mechanisms. Trabecular cells have receptors for corticosteroids and they cause alternation of multiple gene expression leading to the production of extracellular glycosaminoglycans including fibronectin, laminin and collagen. [12] They also decrease the turnover of the extracellular matrix by inhibiting matrix metaloproteinases (MMPs) and tissue plasminogen activator and increasing plasminogen activator inhibitor 1 and tissue inhibitors of MMPs. Therefore, the glycosaminoglycans accumulate in the angle. The corticosteroids also cause inhibition of phagocytosis, proliferation and migration of the trabeculocytes, and formation of certain prostaglandins.

Secondary angle closure glaucoma may occur as chronic and acute forms. In chronic angle closure glaucoma, peripheral anterior synechiae (PAS) develop along the angle. They are being developed due to organization of inflammatory products in the angle. These PAS are broad base, trapezoid and highly pigmented bands that bridge the peripheral iris with the corneal periphery obstructing the angle. They may widen with time, resulting eventually in closure of the angle and increased IOP. Because the angle is progressively closing, the IOP increases gradually without causing an acute stage of increased IOP and without corneal edema. The acute form of angle closure glaucoma occurs secondary to papillary block because of 360° of posterior synechiae. These synechiae develop between the posterior margin of the iris and the crystalline (or intraocular) lens secondary to accumulation of fibrin and inflammatory precipitates over the lens. When the papillary margins are completely blocked, the aqueous humour is trapped in the posterior chamber, accumulates there, resulting in anterior iris displacement (iris bombe). The peripheral iris becomes appositioned against the peripheral cornea and obstructs the angle. The glaucoma in these cases develops abruptly and may be accompanied by ocular pain and corneal edema. A third, rarer mechanism includes the anterior rotation of the lens-iris diaphragm that results in angle closure. The forward rotation is caused by ciliary body and choroidal edema.

3. Uveitic entities associated with glaucoma

3.1. Glaucomatocyclitic crisis (Posner-Schlossman syndrome)

Glaucomatocyclitic crisis is characterized by recurrent episodes of increased IOP and anterior chamber inflammation. Therefore, the uveitis is always accompanied by glaucoma and vice versa. In between, the eye is quiet and the IOP is normal. The disease is usually unilateral and involves the same eye.

Patients complain of blurred or decreased vision and ocular discomfort. Minimal flare and cells (usually +1 or 5-10 cells per wide field magnification of X40) are found in the anterior chamber along with increase in IOP in the range of 40-60mmHg that may reach 70mmHg. Iris heterochromia may appear after recurrent attacks. The first attack is always the most challenging to diagnose. When subsequent episodes occur, the diagnosis is obvious and the patient is aware when they occur. The disease usually appears at the 3rd to 4th decade.

The pathogenesis of the disease is not well established. Viral infection by herpes and cytomegalic viruses, allergic factors and immunogenetic factors related to HLA-Bw54 have been suggested. [13-16] It may also be related to certain prostaglandins such as E released due to vascular incompetence. [17] Indeed, prostaglandin inhibitors, oral indomethacin and subconjunctival polyphloretin, a prostaglandin antagonist have been demonstrated to decrease the IOP. [17], [18]

The disease responds to medical treatment with topical corticosteroid (prednisolone acetate 1% qid) and anti-glaucoma medications such as beta-blockers (timolol 0.5% bid) and carbonic anhydrase inhibitors (acetazolamide 250mg bid or tid). [19] Topical IOP sparing corticosteroids and non-steroidal anti-inflammatory drugs may replace the classic corticosteroids. Prostaglandin inhibitors, oral indomethacin 75-150mg/day and subconjunctival polyphloretin, a prostaglandin antagonist, may also decrease the IOP. No preventive treatment during the remissions is known. In rare cases in which progression in optic disc and visual field damage is demonstrated, trabeculectomy or stenting procedure may be performed. The prognosis is good and some claim that the frequency of the attacks decreaseage. Unfortunately, no prophylactic treatment exists. The risk of developing optic disc and visual field damage is increased with the duration of the disease. Patients with 10 years or more of disease have a risk of 2.8 folds to develop damage than those with duration of less than 10 years.

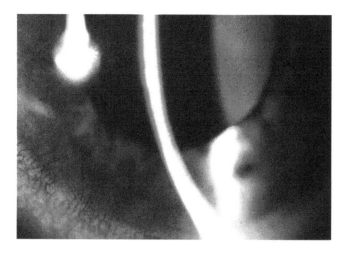

Figure 1. Posner-Schlossman syndrome. Note the few keraticprover the endothelium.

3.2. Fuchs' heterochromic iridocyclitis

The disease is characterized by iris heterochromia and chronic, low-grade iridocyclitis. It appears in the 2nd to 4th decade and is unilateral in 87% of the patients. [20]

The patients may be asymptomatic or may complain of a decrease in vision or change iris color. On examination, heterochromia along with low-grade anterior chamber reaction (flare and cells +1) are noted. Fine keratic precipitates may be noted as well. Secondary open angle glaucoma develops in 13-59% of the patients depending on the duration of the disease. It is more frequent in patients with bilateral disease and in African descends. Posterior subcapsular cataract may also develop.

Treatment for Fuchs' dystrophy without glaucoma is not required since it poorly responds to corticosteroids. The glaucoma may develop late in the course of the disease. Anti-glaucoma medications may be effective initially but later the medical treatment usually fails and filtration surgery is required. [21]

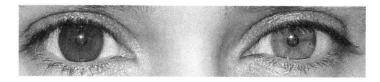

Figure 2. Fuchs' heterochromic iridocyclitis in the right eye. The differential diagnosis for a brighter involved iris is congenital and acquired Horner syndrome (with 2mm ptosis and miosis) and more rarely Posner Schlosmann syndrome and for darker involved iris, siderosis bulbi.

3.3. Glaucoma in juvenile idiopathic arthritic (JIA) uveitis

Secondary glaucoma may develop in 14-42% of the patients with JIA. [22]-[24] The glaucoma is usually open angle. However, papillary block glaucoma and chronic angle closure glaucoma may also develop.

The patient is usually asymptomatic and the eye is quiet. Therefore, any child with pauciarticular arthritis should be referred to ophthalmologic examination every 6 months. If uveitis presents, flare and cells will be present in the anterior segment. In cases of uveitis, measurement of the IOP and evaluation of the optic disc are mandatory. Both the uveitis and glaucoma should be treated early and aggressively. The uveitis is treated in a stepladder manner. The purpose of the treatment is to achieve remission but treatment should be continued even after its achievement. First, topical corticosteroid (prednisolone acetate 1% every 1-2 hours) and cycloplegic (cyclopentholate 1% tid) agent are being used. [25] Change to IOP-sparing or less potent corticosteroids should be performed only when the initial inflammation decreased. If treatment with corticosteroid fails, oral NSAID such as naprosyn (Naproxen®) 5mg/kg twice a day is being used and if this fails, immunosuppressive treatment with oral methotrexate $15mg/m^2$ up to $30mg/m^2$ (or 03-0.5mg/kg) once a week is employed. Common side effects of methotrexate include nausea, anorexia, stomatitis and transient elevation of serum aminotransferase. Alopecia, hematological toxicity, headache, dizziness, fatigue, and mood changes may also occur. A "post-dosing" reaction may occur within 24 hours of receiving methotrexate and is usually characterized by malaise, fatigue, gastrointestinal upset, and occasionally central nervous system manifestations. Liver cirrhosis is a long-term potential complication. Other immunomodulators, such as oral cyclosporine (2-5 mg/kg/day), azathioprine (1-2mg/kg per day), mycophenolate mofetil (300mg/m2 body surface area bid), or chlorambucil (0.10-0.16 mg/kg/day) may be used when methotrexate is not tolerable or when remission is not achieved.

3.4. Sarcoidosis

A multi-organ inflammatory disease that is prevalent in blacks. The patients have pulmonary hilar lymphadenopathy, peripheral lymphadenopathy and cutaneous non-caseating epithelioid granulomas. Ocular involvement occurs in 38% of the patients and may be the first manifestation of the disease. [26] Anterior uveitis is the most common ocular manifestation. At the beginning, the uveitis appears as acute iridocyclitis. A characteristic but not pathognomonicsign is large (mutton fat) keratic precipitates (KPs) over the endothelium. The disease may become chronic and bilateral. The mutton fat PKs are usually encountered at this stage along with Koeppe's nodules on the iris margins and Busacca's nodules on the iris surface. Nodules may also appear in the angle and over the ciliary body. Open angle glaucoma is present in 11%. The usual pathogenesis is obstruction of the angle by inflammatory cells and debris. The disease may mistakenly be considered as Fuchs' heterochromic iridocyclitis. Elevated serum angiotensin converting enzyme or a positive Kveim test will confirm the diagnosis of sarcoid. Additional tests include Gallium [67] scan that shows high intake in the lacrimal and parotid lymph nodes with or without submandibular lymph nodes and serum-lysozyme, which is increased. Treatment includes topical corticosteroid (prednisolone acetate 1% every 1-2 hours) and cycloplegic agent. If the posterior segment is involved, sub-Tenon and or oral corticosteroids (see the section on medical treatment of uveitic glaucoma below) are added. The sub-Tenon injections of corticosteroids may be repeated weekly. However, they should be cautiously used if glaucoma exists. Immunosuppressive agents such as methotrexate should replace corticosteroids if there is no response or contraindications such as steroid-induced glaucoma. In resisting cases, anti-tumor necrosis factor alpha (TNFα) such as infliximab, etanercept, or adalimumab and intravitreal anti-vascular endothelial growth factor such as bevacizumab may be employed. Anti-glaucoma medications are indicated. Generally, the long-term prognosis is poor.

3.5. Herpetic keratouveitic glaucoma

Secondary open angle glaucoma may develop in herpetic keratouveitis in 10-54%. [27], [28] The disease appears weeks to years after recurrent episodes of keratouveitis with either stromal keratitis (96%) or metaherpetic ulcer (4%). The pathogenesis is probably a complex of direct injury to the trabeculocytes by the virus, inflammatory products and response to corticosteroids. The condition is responsive to medical treatment with topical corticosteroid and antiglaucoma medications such as β-blockers, α-agonists and topical and oral carbonic anhydrase inhibitors. In patients with several episodes of keratouveitis in a year, oral acyclovir 400 mg bid for a year or more may decrease the recurrences.

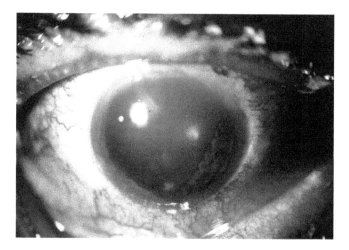

Figure 3. Glaucoma in herpetic keratouveitis. Note the mild stromal haze from stromal keratitis and posterior synechia.

3.6. Congenital rubella

Congenital rubella affects the heart, auditory system and the eye. It may cause cataract, retinopathy, glaucoma and microphthalmia in 30-60% of the affected children. Glaucoma appears in 2-15% and is frequently associated with cataract and microphthalmia. [29] The pathogenesis is multi-factorial. Congenital angle abnormalities, chronic iridocyclitis, papillary block and angle closure glaucoma from intumescent cataract or microphthalmia are implicated. The glaucoma may appear at any age and therefore routine follow-up that includes measurement of the IOP and evaluation of the optic disc is required for lifetime. It should be performed at least every 6 months. If glaucoma is diagnosed, treatment should be aggressive and follow-up should be frequent to prevent blindness since it may occur in 44%. A peripheral iridectomy should be performed if cataract surgery is performed to deepen the anterior chamber and to prevent papillary block glaucoma.

3.7. Glaucoma in idiopathic uveitis

Any patient with chronic or recurrent anterior uveitis from unknown cause may develop glaucoma. Thus, in all patients with chronic or recurrent uveitis, IOP measurements should be obtained. Independently, medical treatment for the uveitis and for the glaucoma should be initiated to achieve remission of the inflammation and control the IOP.

3.8. Phacoanaphylactic uveitis (phacoantigenic uveitis)

Phacoanaphylaxis is a granulomatous uveitis from liberated crystalline lens proteins and contact with blood circulation. This disorder may be classified also as part of the lens-induced glaucomas. [30] It is the result of cataract extraction or traumatic lens rupture. The disorder may occur any time after surgery or trauma. It may occur spontaneously usually in microphthalmic eyes. It is type III hypersensitivity (immune complex). It usually causes hypotony and rarely pupillary block glaucoma or angle closure glaucoma from peripheral anterior synechiae. Keratic precipitates may appear on the cornea and the intraocular lens (IOL), hypopion and numerous white cells in the anterior chamber and vitreous may be present. Remnants of the crystalline lens are always present, while cultures are negative. Anterior chamber tap reveals foamy macrophages (as seen in phacolytic glaucoma). A high suspicion index is required because the disease may be similar to infectious endophthalmitis (but without pain), sterile endophthalmitis and toxic anterior chamber reaction (fibrinoid reaction). The respond to corticosteroids is temporary and removal of the lens remnants is the treatment of choice.

3.9. Uveitis-glaucoma-hyphema (UGH) syndrome

Uveitis-glaucoma-hyphema (UGH) syndrome is a triad classically caused by subluxated or mal-positioned IOL (usually an anterior chamber IOL) rubbing against the iris and causing release of pigment and bleeding that result in open angle glaucoma. [31] If vitreous hemorrhage also presents, the condition is called UGH plus. Incomplete UGH is when uveitis and sometimes glaucoma are absent. The condition may also be caused by excessive movement of a small IOL. The patient complaints are sudden (within minutes to hours) decrease in vision that gradually improves over hours to days, and sometimes, ocular pain. The patient may describe his vision as "white-out" or having reddish tint (erythropsia). The condition occurs from one week to months after surgery. It is diagnosed by attacks of this triad and the presence of iris transillumination corresponding to the rubbing site. The diagnosis is easiest during the attack. A blood cloth or hyphema may be observed. The diagnosis can be confirmed by ultrasound biomicroscopy (UBM) and anterior segment optical coherence tomography (AS-OCT) showing a contact between the optic or haptic and the iris. The complications include pseudophakic bullous keratopathy, corneal staining and cystoid macular edema (CME). The differential diagnosis includes amaurosis fugax and vertebrobasilar insufficiency. Amaurosis fugax occurs more rapidly (within seconds to minutes) and loss of light perception in at least one quadrant. Loss of light perception never occurs in UGH syndrome and there is always a history of cataract extraction and IOL implantation or iris device implantation. The differentiation between the two is crucial because patients with amaurosis fugax may be treated with anti-coagulants that may increase the bleeding in UGH syndrome. Patients may respond to topical corticosteroids and anti-glaucoma medications. The definite treatment of UGH is replacement or repositioning of the IOL.

4. Other uveitic glaucomas

Glaucoma has been reported in patients with pars planitis (8%), uveitic from Reiter's syndrome (1%), ankylosing spondylitis, hemorrhagic fever with renal syndrome (nephropathia epidemica) and epidemic dropsy from ingestion of sanguinarine in Argemone mexicana oil. Bilateral acute angle closure glaucoma due to uveal effusion has been described in acquired immunodeficiency syndrome (AIDS) and responded to medical treatment with cycloplegics, topical corticosteroids and anti-glaucoma medications. [32]

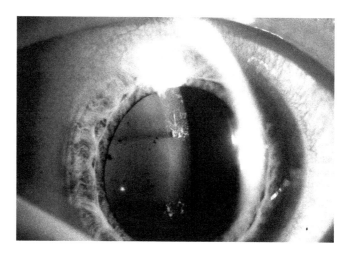

Figure 4. Reiter's syndrome. Note the pigment over the crystalline lens after pupil dilation and release of posterior synechiae.

5. Diagnosis

Patients with acute closed-angle glaucoma may present with ocular and brow ace, blurred vision, halos, photophobia and even nausea and vomiting. Patients with open or chronic angle closure glaucoma are asymptomatic.

All uveitis patients should be routinely evaluated for IOP, which is elevated (>21mmHg) in uveitic glaucoma. In acute closed angle glaucoma, the cornea may be edematous and ciliary and conjunctival congestion may be present. Gonioscopy should be performed to define the type of glaucoma. Topical glycerin 50-100% would clear corneal edema for evaluating the angle and posterior segment. Otherwise, the corneal epithelium may be removed with a blade or 70% alcohol on a cotton-tipped applicator. If the cornea is still cloud, UBM or AS-OCT may replace gonioscopy in evaluating is performed the angle. Optic disc evaluation by slit lamp biomicroscopy and other imaging techniques (OCT, scanning laser polarimetry (GDx) or Heidelberg retinal tomography (HRT)) when the cornea is clear. Visual fields should be obtained in patients with cup/disc ratio of 0.6 or more for baseline and follow-up documentation of the progression of the glaucoma. In patients with cup/disc ratio of less than 0.6, the visual field is usually normal. The visual field may be abnormal due to CME (central relative scotoma) and retinitis or retinal scarring (defects corresponding to these areas). CME and macular atrophy may be confirmed by OCT. Differentiation should be made between steroid responder (the IOP returns to normal upon discontinuation of the corticosteroids) and corticosteroid-induced glaucoma (the IOP remains high). Differentiation between increased IOP due to increased inflammation and steroid responder may be performed by replacing the corticosteroids with IOP-sparing corticosteroids. The IOP should decrease.

6. Medical treatment

Treatment is aimed to control both the uveitis and IOP. The uveitis is treated by topical and/or systemic corticosteroids and/ or immunosuppressive drugs to achieve resolution or remission. Sub-Tenon corticosteroids such as triamcinolone acetonid (Kenalog®) 20-40mg (0.5-1ml) or methylprednisolone acetate (Depo-medrol®) 40-80mg may be given to treat noninfectious uveitis and macular edema. Intravitreal implants such as Ozurdex®, a copolymer of glycolic and lactic acid with 700μg of dexamethasone may be injected through the pars plana with 22G injector. It dissolves gradually over 6 months to H_2O and CO_2 and releases the dexamethasone. However, they all and especially those that cannot be removed (sub-Tenonand intravitreal) should be used cautiously in patients with glaucoma and are contraindicated in steroid responders and steroid-induced glaucoma. In cases of steroid responders orcorticosteroid-induced glaucoma, topical corticosteroids may be replaced by IOP-sparing corticosteroids such as such as loteprednol etabonate 0.5% (Lotemax®) or rimexolone 1%(Vexol®) but because of low potency, they may be more frequently required. These agents are especially useful for maintenance. Alternatively, topical non-steroidal anti-inflammatory (NSAID) such as nepafenac 0.1% (Nevanac®), ketorolac tromethamine 0.5% (Acular® or Tradol®), diclofenac sodium (Voltaren® (0.1%), Solaraze® (3%)) or indometha-cin 1% (Indoptic®) may be used. Topical immunosuppressive agent such as cyclosporine A 0.5-2% and systemic immunosuppressive drugs may be alternatives for corticosteroids and NSAID. The dosage of corticosteroids depends on the severity of inflammation and is titrat-ed according to the response to treatment. The corticosteroids are gradually tapered accord-ing to the response since abrupt discontinuation may cause flare-up. Topical cycloplegic agents such as cyclopentholate HCl 1% (in neonates 0.5%) tid are added to control pain that originates from the ciliary body and to prevent the formation of posterior synechiae.

The preferred anti-glaucoma medications include topical alpha agonists, carbonic anhydrase inhibitors and beta-blockers. Prostaglandins may be added in a quiet eye but should be avoided in an inflamed eye and herpetic keratouveitis because they may exacerbate the in-traocular inflammation and cause CME. [33]- [35] Oral or intravenous carbonic anhydrase inhibitors (acetazolamide 500mg) and hyperosmotic agents (oral glycerol 50% or IV manni-tol 20% 1gr/kg) should be added if the reduction in IOP is not to the normal range. The effi-cacy of prostaglandins and alpha adrenergic agonists may decrease with concurrent use of topical or systemic NSAID. [36], [37] The glaucoma is controlled by medical treatment in 26% of the children and 24% of the adults. [6] In near future, ocular implants containing slow release IOP sparing corticosteroids may improve the visual outcome of patients with macular edema secondary to uveitis without inducing steroid-induced glaucoma. In future, new drugs such as Rho kinase inhibitors may replace existing medications.

7. Laser treatment

7.1. Laser iridotomy

Laser iridotomy is indicated for all cases of secondary papillary block glaucoma, chronic an-gle closure glaucoma and prophylactically when progressive anterior synechiae are being formed. [38] It is performed either to allow aqueous humour access into the anterior cham-ber in papillary block glaucoma or increase in the depth of the anterior chamber in chronic angle closure glaucoma. In some cases of papillary block glaucoma, the glaucoma may not resolve because the entrapment of aqueous in several compartments behind the iris. In such cases, more than one iridotomy is required.

The first treatment modality, which is usually the simplest, if the cornea is clear, is peripher-al laser iridotomy. It is usually performed with Neodymium: Yttrium-Aluminum-Garnet (Nd:YAG) laser. Topical glycerin may be placed over the cornea before the procedure if it is edematous. After instillation of topical pilocarpine 2% or 4% and topical analgesic (e.g., oxy-buprocaine HCl 0.4% or proparacaine HCl 0.5%) eye drop, a spot of 10mJ is placed over the peripheral iris. Two pulses may be used simultaneously. The size of the spot is constant de-pending on the instrument (50-70μm). The spot is placed at the periphery of the iris in the superior half to avoid glare, and over a thin part of the iris (usually a crypt) avoiding blood vessels. If bleeding occurs, the cornea is pressed by a contact lens until bleeding ceases. The procedure may be performed with contact lens such as Abraham (+66D), Wise (+103D), CGIor without it. The advantages of a contact lens are additional magnification, focusing the beam, absorbing part of the heat, stabilizing the eye and keeping the eyelids open. Topical apraclonidine (Iopidine®) 0.5%-1.0% or other alpha 2 agonist (e.g., brimonidine tartrate) is administered following the procedure to decrease IOP spikes and corticosteroids such as prednisolone acetate 1% qid are prescribed for a week to decrease intraocular inflammation and risk of synechiae formation. Additional anti-glaucoma medications may be added. This procedure facilitates aqueous flow from the posterior into the anterior chamber and may result in deepening of the anterior chamber and lowering the IOP. The major complication is acceleration of cataract. If Nd:YAG laser is unavailable, Argon laser iridotomy may be performed. The parameters for this procedure depend on the iris pigmentation. For brighter iris, the power is lower than for darker ones. The preparatory stretch burns are of 200-600mW, 0.2-0.6 sec, 200-500 μ m. The penetration burns are of 800-1000mW, 0.2 sec, 50μm. The iridotomy size should be increased to 150-500μm. The position of the Argon iridotomy in this case is preferably supero-nasal to prevent injury to the macula. Argon laser may increase the intraocular inflammation because it releases pigment due to a different mechanism of action (plasma creation by ionizing in cases of ND:YAG versus coagulation in Argon). The treatment before and after the procedure is identical to Nd:YAG laser iridotomy. Perforation of the iris is confirmed when aqueous mixed with pigment is flowing from the posterior to the anterior chamber through the iridotomy. The lens should be visible through the iridotomy, since positive transillumination is not reliable. When laser iridotomy is not feasible or is impossible to perform, surgical peripheral iridectomy should be performed. Complications include visual disturbances such as halo and glare, development and progression of cataract, transient corneal burns, temporary increase in IOP, intraocular inflammation and rarely retinal injury, CME and malignant glaucoma.

Argon laser trabeculoplasty has no role in uveitic open-angle glaucoma because of its low success rate. It may increase the intraocular inflammation and alter the angle structure. Some authors found selective (ND:YAG) laser trabeculoplasty to be effective in 20% of the patients, [39] but the follow-up was limited and the effectiveness is expected to decline. Therefore, it is not an ideal solution. The reason is that both procedures do not prevent the obstruction of the open angle by inflammatory products.

7.2. Surgical treatment

Surgical procedures are reserved for patients who fail to respond to medical treatment. Surgical intervention is required in 56% of the children and in 35% of the adults with uveitic glaucoma. [6] Any intraocular intervention should be performed on a quiet eye for at least 3 months. Topical corticosteroids or other medications as indicated above should be administrated two weeks preoperatively and postoperatively to control the uveitis. Systemic corticosteroids may be added. Any intervention on an inflamed eye may result in exacerbation of the uveitis, failure of the procedure and complications. When increased postoperative intraocular inflammation is anticipated, enoxaparin (Clexan®) (40mg/500 balanced salt solution (BSS)), a low-weight molecular heparin decreases the intensity of such inflammation in surgery for uveitic eyes as it does in congenital cataract surgery. [40] Glaucoma surgery may be combined with cataract extraction. The data on the newer procedures in uveitic glaucoma are limited. Detailed description of the newer devices can be found in chapter 19 in this book, chapter 20 in Rumelt S. Ed. Glaucoma – basic and clinical concepts. Rijeka, Croatia: Intech 2011 and chapter 17 in Rumelt S. Ed. Advances in ophthalmology. Rijeka, Croatia: Intech 2012.

7.3. Trabeculectomy

As for all secondary glaucomas, uveitic glaucoma that does not respond to medical treatment should be treated with trabeculectomy and mitomycin C (MMC) or other shunting procedure. [41]-[46] Without MMC, trabeculectomy may fail. Trabeculectomy with MMC is indicated for open and closed angle glaucomas. MMC decreases the risk of scarring of the filtering bleb, which is higher in uveitic glaucoma than in primary glaucomas, because of the increased postoperative inflammation. MMC 0.04% may be applied for 3 min under the scleral flap (or the conjunctiva) avoiding the conjunctival margins. Copious BSS irrigation is performed to remove the free MMC.

The cumulative probability for success of trabeculectomy with MMC or 5-fluorouracil at 1 and 2 years was 78 and 68% respectively. [4] Risk factors for failure include male gender and young age. [47] The use of spacers such as collagen matrix (Ologen®) or other biodegradable material may prove to be beneficial as well as injection of subconjunctival bevacizumab 2.5mg/0.1ml.These should be evaluated for uveitic glaucoma.

8. Non-Penetrating Glaucoma Surgery (NPGS)

Non-penetrating glaucoma surgery (NPGS) is a filtration procedure in which the anterior chamber is not penetrated. [48]- [50] It is based on creation of a partial thickness scleral flap and a deep pocket in the area of the outer wall of the Schlemm's canal. It involves the Schlemm's canal without penetrating its inner wall. Three variations of the procedure exist: canaloplasty, viscocanalostomy and deep sclerostomy. In the first procedure, a 10-0 nylon is passed through the Schlemm's canal while in the second, viscoelastic agent such as hyaluronic acid (Healon®) is injected into the canal. The aqueous flows through the trabeculo-Descemet's membrane into scleral pocket and from there to surrounding blood and aqueous vessels. The NPGS with intraoperative MMC is promising showing good short-term (between one and three years) success, but a long follow-up is required.

9. Glaucoma drainage implants

Drainage implants drain the aqueous humour to the subconjunctival space. They are considered if one or two trabeculectomies with MMC fail or if extensive conjunctival scarring exists. [51] Some authors who have favorable outcomes with glaucoma drainage implant select it as the procedure of choice in uveitic glaucoma. [52], [53] Two types of drainage implants exist. The first type is with control of the flow (with a "valve" or flow resistance) and includes Ahmed (New World Medical, Rancho Cucamonga, CA) and Krupin-Denver (Hood Laboratories, Pembroke, MA) drainage implants. The second type is without pressure control (no valve) and includes Molteno single or double plate (IOP, Inc., Costa Mesa, CA, USA, and Molteno OpLimited, Dunedin, New Zealand), Baerveldt (Advanced Medical Optics, Santa Ana, California, USA), Shocket (self-assembled) and Eagle Vision (Eagle Vision, Inc. Memphis, TN, USA) implants. The later require blocking the aqueous flow for a few days externally by temporary suture or internally passing a suture through the lumen of the tube or injecting viscoelastic agent. The implantation may also be performed as a two-stage implantation, to decrease the risk for postoperative hypotony. Ahmed and Krupin implants should be preferred over the implants without a valve, because the risk for postoperative overflow and hypotony that may result in endothelial-iris and lens touch. This is more prevalent in patients with uveitis than without it because the aqueous production is usually low. Ahmed valve has convenient plate of variable sizes including for pediatric population.

The success rate of Ahmed implant in uveitic glaucoma at one year is 77-94% and at 4 years 50%. [54]- [56] The success rate of Baeveldt implant at 1 year is 92%. [47] A decrease in corneal endothelial cell count has been observed with glaucoma drainage devices (Ahmed) in comparison with non-valved implanted eyes. The decrease in endothelium is related to the age of the patient, duration of the uveitis and presence of the implant and corneal-valve touch. [57]

9.1. ExPress shunt

It is expected that this device will have the advantages of trabeculectomy (guarded filtration) and other glaucoma drainage device (uniform internal opening) as long as it will not be blocked by inflammatory products. We have found that it is beneficial in secondary glaucomas including uveitic glaucoma (in publication). The only exceptions are neovascular glaucoma and iridocorneal endothelial syndrome where it usually fails. No other data are available on the outcome of ExPress implantation in uveitic glaucoma.

9.2. IStent

IStent is a titanium device that is placed into the Schlemm's canal through the anterior chamber. This device may be effective in secondary glaucoma and may decrease the requirement for postoperative hypotensive medications. It has not been proven yet to be effective in uveitic glaucoma.

9.3. Trabectome

Trabectome is a micro-electrical device that removes the trabecular meshwork and unroof the Schlemm's canal under gonioscopy to decrease the resistance to aqueous outflow. No results of this device in uveitic glaucoma are available. It is expected that it will have only a

temporary effect if the uveitis persists, since new inflammatory products may gradually obstruct the surgical site.

9.4. Solx Gold shunt and CyPass

These devises are placed into the suprachoroidal space. Based on other devises with similar
principle, it is expected that these devices will fail due to obstruction by uveal tissue especially in eyes with uveitis.

9.5. Cycloablation

Cycloablation, preferably with 810nm infrared diode laser may be applied in uncontrolled
glaucoma with no potential for improvement in visual acuity in which other anti-glaucoma
procedures failed. [58], [59] The reason is that it is difficult to predict the outcome of the
treatment (final IOP) and to control the post-treatment intraocular inflammation, which is
usually, exacerbate. Such inflammation may result in CME with decrease in visual acuity
and central scotoma, papillary and retropupillary membranes and phthisis bulbi. The initial
settings for trans-scleral cyclophotocoagulation with this laser is 1,250mW, 2sec. Following
topical anesthesia and additional peribulbar lidocaine 2% 2ml, the probe is placed 1.2mmbe-
hind the limbus. The power is increased in 150mW increments but not over 2250mW until a
"pop" sound is heard. Then it is decreased in 150mW until no "pop" is heard and treatment
begins. Eighteen spots are delivered to 270° avoiding 3:00 and 9:00 positions where the long
posterior ciliary nerves enter the eye. Prevention of CME may be possible by topical NSAID
such as diclofenac sodium (Voltaren®) 0.1% qid for 6 months. Decrease in visual acuity
mayoccur from CME if prophylactic treatment is refrained or in cases of advanced visual
field loss (splitting of the fixation or high mean deviation) as in other surgical procedures.

10. Follow-up

The follow-up intervals depend on the severity of the uveitis and glaucoma. Patients with
quiet eyes and controlled IOP should be observed at least every 6 months. If the uveitis is
active or the glaucoma is uncontrolled, the follow-up interval should be decreased. The follow-up examinations include IOP measurement, complete anterior and posterior segments
for activity of the uveitis, optic disc cupping and other means as necessary (e.g., visual fields
and OCT).

11. Prognosis

The prognosis depends on the etiology of the uveitis and severity of the inflammation and
the glaucoma. Early medical and surgical interventions may improve the visual outcome
and obtain resolution or long-term remission of the uveitis.

12. Summary

Uveitic glaucoma is a heterogeneous group of diseases in which glaucoma develops secondary to uveitis. The diagnosis is based on elevated IOP. Periodic evaluation of the optic disc should be made, and in patients with cup/disc ratio of 0.6 or more, visual field evaluations should be obtained. The management includes treating the uveitis, glaucoma and the underlying disorder. Most of the uveitis types should be treated although uveitis in juvenile rheumatoid arthritis requires minimal medical treatment to obtain remission and the uveitis in Fuchs' heterochromic iridocyclitis does not require any treatment. In contrary, glaucoma should always be treated aggressively. If medical treatment for glaucoma fails, surgical intervention should be promptly applied. Evaluation of the newer procedures and implants is required to determine the best approach.

Author details

Shimon Rumelt

Department of Ophthalmology, Western Galilee, Nahariya Medical Center, Nahariya, Israel

References

[1] Foster CS, Vitale AT. Diagnosis and treatment of uveitis. Philadelphia: WB Sounders. 2001:17-23.

[2] Vadot E. Epidemiology of intermediate uveitis: a prospective study in Savoy. Dev Ophthalmol 1992;23:33-4.

[3] Gritz C, Wong G. Incidence and prevalence of uveitis in Northern California. The Northern California Epidemiology of Uveitis Study. Ophthalmology 2004;111:491-500.

[4] Merayo-Lloves J, Power WJ, Rodriguez A et al. Secondary glaucoma in patients with uveitis. Ophthalmologica 1999;213:300-4.

[5] Takahashi T, Ohtani S, Miyata K et al. Clinical evaluation of uveitis-associated secondary glaucoma. Jpn J Ophthalmol 2002;46:556-62.

[6] Heinz C, Koch JM, Zurek-Imhoff B, Heiligenhaus A. Prevalence of uveitic secondary glaucoma and success of nonsurgical treatment in adults and children in a tertiary referral center. Ocul Immunol Inflamm 2009;17:243-8.

[7] Netland PA, Denton NC. Uveitic glaucoma. Contemp Ophthalmol 2006;5:1-26.

[8] Jha P, Bora PS, Bora NS. Role of complement in ocular immune response. In: Drat DA, Dana R, D'amore P, Niederkorn JY. Immunology, inflammation and diseases of the eye. Oxford, UK: Academic Press. 2011:37.

[9] Rao PV, Deng P, Maddala R, Epstein DL, Li CY, Shimokawa H. Expression of dominant negative Rho-binding domain of Rho-kinase in organ cultured human eye anterior segments increases aqueous humor outflow. Mol Vis 2005;27:288-97.

[10] Pattabiraman PP, Rao PV. Mechanistic basis of Rho GTPase-induced extracellular matrix synthesis in trabecular meshwork cells. Am J Physiol Cell Physiol 2010;298:C749-63.

[11] Becker B. Intraocular pressure response to topical corticosteroids. Invest Ophthalmol Vis Sci 1965;4:198-205.

[12] Tektas OY, Heinz C, Heiligenhaus A, Hammer CM, Luetjen-Drecoll E. Morphological changes of trabeculectomy specimens in different kinds of uveitic glaucoma. Curr Eye Res 2011;36:442-

[13] Hirose S, Ohno S, Masuda H. HLA Bw54 and glaucomatocyclitic crisis. Arch Ophthalmol 1985;103:1837-9.

[14] Bloch ME, Dussaix E, Sibillat M. Posner Schlossman syndrome. A cytomregalovirus infection? Bull Soc Ophthalmol Fr 1998;8:75-6.

[15] Yamanto S, Langston PD, Tada R. Possible role of herpes simplex virus in Posner Schlossman syndrome. Am J Ophthalmol 1995;119:796-8.

[16] Knox DL. Glaucomatocyclitic crises and systemic disease: peptic ulcer, other gastrointestinal disorder, various allergies and stress. Trans Am Ophthalmol Soc 1988;86:473-95.

[17] Matsuda K, Izawa Y, Mishima S. Prostaglandins and glaucomatocyclitic crisis. Jpn J Ophthalmol 1975;19:368-75.

[18] Hong C, Song KY. Effect of apraclonidine hydrochloride on the attack of Posner Schlossman syndrome. Korean J Ophthalmol 1993;7:28-33.

[19] Chandler M, Grant WM. In: Lectures on glaucoma. Philadelphia: Lea & Febiger. 1954. p. 257.

[20] Kimura SJ, Hogan MJ, Thygeson P. Fuchs' syndrome of heterochromic cyclitis. AMA Arch Ophthalmol 1955;54:179-86.

[21] Liesegang T. Clinical features and prognosis in Fuchs' uveitis syndrome. Arch Ophthalmol 1982;100:1622-6.

[22] Key SN III, Kimura SJ. Iridocyclitis associated with juvenile rheumatoid arthritis. Am J Ophthalmol 1975;80:425-29.

[23] Kanski JJ, Shun-Shin GA. Systemic uveitis syndromes in childhood: An analysis of 340 cases. Ophthalmology 1984;91:1247-52.

[24] Wolf MD, Lichter PR, Ragsdale CG. Prognostic factors in the uveitis of juvenile rheumatoid arthritis. Ophthalmology 1987;94:1242-6.

[25] Foster CS, Havrlikova K, Baltatzis S et al. Secondary glaucoma in patients with juvenile rheumatoid arthritis-associated iridocyclitis. ACTA Ophthalmol Scand 2000;78:576-9.

[26] Oebenauf CD, Shaw HE, Sydnor CF et al. Sarcoidosis and its ophthalmic manifestations. Am J Ophthalmol 1978;86:648-55.

[27] Karbassi M, Raizman MB, Schuman JS. Herpes zoster ophthalmicus. Surv Ophthalmol 1992;36:395-410.

[28] Miserocchi , Waheed NK, Dios E et al. Visual outcome in herpes simplex virus and varicella zoster virus uveitis: a clinical evaluation and comparison. Ophthalmology 2002;109:1532-7.

[29] Boniuk M. Glaucoma in congenital rubella syndrome. Int Ophthalmol Clin 1972;12:121-6.

[30] Marak GE Jr. Phaendophthalmitis. Surv Ophthalmol 1992;36:325-39.

[31] van Oye R, Gelisken O. Pseudophakic glaucoma. Int Ophthalmol 1985;8:183-6.

[32] Nash RW, Lindquist TD. Bilateral angle-closure glaucoma associated with uveal effusion: presenting sign of HIV infection. Surv Ophthalmol 1992;36:255-8.

[33] Fechtner RD, Khouri AS, Zimmerman TJ et al. Anterior uveitis associated with latanoprost. Am J Ophthalmol 1998;126:37-41.

[34] Smith SL, Pruitt CA, Sine CS et al. Latanoprost 0.005% and anterior segment uveitis. ACTA Ophthalmol Scand 1999;77:668-72.

[35] Fortuna E, Cervantes-Castaneda RA, Bhat P et al. Flare-up rates with bimatoprost therapy in uveitic glaucoma. Am J Ophthalmol 2008;146:876-82.

[36] Sponsel WE, Paris G, Trigo Y et al. Latanoprost and brimonidine: therapeutic and physiologic assessment before and after oral non-steroidal anti-inflammatory therapy. Am J Ophthalmol 2002;133:11-18.

[37] Kahsiwagi K, Tsukahara S. Effect of non-steroidal anti-inflammatory ophthalmic solution on intraocular pressure reduction by latanoprost. Br J Ophthalmol 2003;87:297-301.

[38] Spencer NA, Hall AJ, Stawell RJ. Nd:YAG laser iridotomy in uveitic glaucoma. Clin Experiment Ophthalmol 2001;29:217-9.

[39] Siddique SS, Suelves AM, Baheti U, Foster CS. Glaucoma and uveitis. Surv Ophthalmol 2013;58:1-10.

[40] Rumelt S, Stolovich C, Segal ZI, et al. Intraoperative enoxaparin minimizes inflammatory reaction after pediatric cataract surgery. Am J Ophthalmol 2006;141:433-437.

[41] Hoskins HD Jr, Hetherington J Jr, Shaffer RN. Surgical management of inflammatory glaucomas. Perspectives in Ophthalmology 1977;1:173-81.

[42] Patitsas C, RockwEJ, Meisler DM al. Glaucoma filtering surgery with postoperative 5-fluorouracil in patients with intraocular inflammatory disease. Ophthalmology 1992;99:594-9.

[43] Prata JA Jr, Neves RA, Minckler DS et al. Trabeculectomy with mitomycin C in glaucoma associated with uveitis. Ophthalmic Surg 1994;25:616-20.

[44] Towler HM, Bates AK, Broadway DC et al. Primary trabeculectomy with 5-fluorouracil for glaucoma secondary to uveitis. Ocular Immunol Inflamm 1995;3:163-70.

[45] Wright MM, McGehee RF, Pederson JE. Intraoperative mitomycin C for glaucoma associated with ocular inflammation. Ophthalmic Surg Lasers 1997;28:370-6.

[46] Yalvac IS, Sungur G, Turhan E et al. Trabeculectomy with mitomycin C in uveitic glaucoma associated with Biet disease. J Glaucoma 2004;13:450-3.

[47] Ceballos EM, Beck AD, Lynn MJ. Trabeculectomy with antiproliferative agents in uveitic glaucoma. J Glaucoma 2002;11:189-96.

[48] Souissi K, El Afrit MA, Trojet S, Kraiem A. Deep sclerectomy for the management of uveitic glaucoma. J Fr Ophtalmol 2006;29:265-8.

[49] Auer C, Mermoud A, Herbort CP. Deep sclerectomy for the management of uncontrolled uveitic glaucoma: preliminary data. Klin Monbl Augenheilkd 2004;221:339-42.

[50] Anand N. Deep sclerectomy with mitomycin C for glaucoma secondary to uveitis. Eur J Ophthalmol 2011;21:708-14.

[51] Chow K, Mora J. Preferences for glaucoma drainage device implantation and cyclodestruction in Australia and New Zealand. J Glaucoma 2012;21:199-205.

[52] Vuori ML. Molteno aqueous shunt as a primary surgical intervention for uveitic glaucoma: long-term results. Acta Ophthalmol 2010;88:33-6.

[53] Hill RA, Nguyen QH, Baerveldt G et al. Trabeculectomy and Molteno implantation for glaucomas associated with uveitis. Ophthalmology 1993;100:903-8.

[54] Gil-Carrasco F, Salinas-Van Orman E, Recillas-Gispert C et al. Ahmed valve implant for uncontrolled uveitic glaucoma. Ocular Immunol Inflamm 1998;6:27-37.

[55] Da Mata A, Burk SE, Netland PA et al. Management of uveitic glaucoma with Ahmed glaucoma valve implantation. Ophthalmology 1999;106:2168-72.

[56] Papadaki TG, Acharopoulos IP, Pasquale LR et al. Long-term results of Ahmed glau-coma valve implantation for uveitic glaucoma. Am J Ophthalmol 2007;144:62-9.

[57] Kalinina Ayuso V, Scheerlinck LM, de Boer JH. The Effect of an Ahmed glaucoma valve implant on corneal endothelial cell density in children with glaucoma secondary to uveitis. Am J Ophthalmol 2012, in press.

[58] Sung VC, Barton K. Management of glaucomas. Curr Opin Ophthalmol 2004 ; 15:136-40.

[59] Kuchtey RW, Lowder CY, Smith SD. Glaucoma in patients with ocular inflammatory disease. Ophthalmol Clin North Am 2005;18:421-30.

Chapter 2

Neovascular Glaucoma

Cynthia Esponda-Lammoglia,
Rafael Castaneda-Díez, Gerardo García-Aguirre,
Oscar Albis-Donado and Jesús Jiménez-Román

Additional information is available at the end of the chapter

1. Introduction

Iris neovascularization and angle closure glaucoma are serious complications of a number of diseases affecting the eye. Pathologic intraocular neovascularization can be potentially blinding if not detected and treated promptly.

The first report of neovascular glaucoma was made in 1871. It was described as a condition in which the eye developed progressive neovascularization of the iris and lens, elevated intraocular pressure and blindness. First called hemorrhagic glaucoma because of its association with bleeding of the anterior chamber, it has also been called congestive glaucoma, rubeotic glaucoma and diabetic hemorrhagic glaucoma.

During the first descriptions of this type of glaucoma, only clinical findings were mentioned, but in 1906, Coats, described the histological findings of new vessels on the iris of an eye with a history of central retinal vein occlusion. In 1928, Salus, described new vessels on the irises of diabetic patients. In 1937, with the introduction of clinical gonioscopy, the new vessels found in the angle and the histological findings were correlated, explaining the mechanism of angle closure, and in 1963, Weiss and colleagues, proposed the term neovascular glaucoma, which includes the real cause of the rise in intraocular pressure.

2. Etiology

There are many systemic disease and ocular conditions that cause neovascular glaucoma, but they all share a common etiology, which is retinal ischemia, and hypoxia that triggers a pro-angiogenic cascade that finally causes the growth of defective vessels with altered permeability. There are three common causes of NVG: Proliferative diabetic retinopathy, central retinal vein occlusion and ocular ischemic syndrome.

2.1. Common causes

2.1.1. Proliferative diabetic retinopathy

Neovascular Glaucoma is a late manifestation of proliferative diabetic retinopathy (PDR), although it may occur due to ischemia, before neovascularization of the retina or optic disc are present, the most common presentation is in association with PDR. The time of progression from iris neovascularization (IN) to neovascular glaucoma (NVG) is not well established because in some cases it progresses very rapidly, in others it might remain stable for years or even regress with treatment.

The reported rate of IN is 1-10% among all diabetics and about 64% among patients with PDR. Prevalence of NVG in DM is 2%, but it increases to 21% in PDR where the frequency of IN can be as high as 65%. All of these risk factors plus activation of the inflammation cascade by ocular surgery makes the incidence of NVG, rise to 80%, in eyes after pars plana vitrectomy.

NVG is caused more frequently by diabetes than by retinal vein occlusions in Mexico. The proportion is precisely the opposite as that reported in a classic work (Brown et al. 1984). We found that 114 out of 134 (85%) patients operated with an Ahmed valve for NVG during a 22-month period were diabetic (Albis-Donado et al. 2012).

2.1.2. Central retinal vein occlusion

One third of the central retinal vein occlusion (CRVO) cases are ischemic at presentation, the remaining two thirds are non-ischemic, but with a conversion to ischemic rate of about 10%. NVG is a frequent complication of ischemic central retinal vein occlusion. The larger the area of capillary non-perfusion, the greater the risk of developing NVG, especially during the first 18 months.

In general, the development of NVG in CRVO depends upon the severity and extent of the ischemia, for example, hemi retinal vein occlusion or branch retinal vein occlusion have a lower risk of developing NVG and in either case, only if ischemic. Studies have indicated that at least half of the retina must be ischemic for NVG to develop.

In cases in which the ischemic subtype was not defined, the incidence of NVG at 6 months after the CRVO was 50%. In cases of non-ischemic CRVO, the incidence of NVG was approximately 1% eight to fifteen months after the event. NVG incidence in ischemic CRVO ranged from 23% to 60%, but it has been reported to be as high as 80% over a period of 12 to 15 months.

2.1.3. Ocular ischemic syndrome

Ocular ischemic syndrome is caused by reduced blood flow to the eye, which produces anterior and posterior segment ischemia, resulting in the development of iris and angle neovascularization. This is caused by severe carotid artery occlusion (greater than 90%), occlusive disease of the aortic arch or the ophthalmic artery, and less frequently when the ciliary arteries are involved.

2.2. Uncommon causes

2.2.1. Ocular tumors

The development of NVG has been reported in several ocular tumors such as melanoma, choroidal hemangioma, retinoblastoma, malignant lymphoma and some metastatic tumors. Radiation retinopathy after the treatment of certain tumors has been associated with the development of NVG because irradiation causes retinal capillary non-perfusion and retinal ischemia.

2.2.2. Uveitis

NVG has been reported in both anterior and posterior uveitis. It is thought that inflammation and its related Inflammatory factors may directly cause neovascularization on the iris, angle and retina.

Diseases Associated With Retinal Neovascularization
Diabetes mellitus*
Age-related macular degeneration*
Retinopathy of prematurity*
Central retinal vein occlusion* Branch retinal vein occlusion*
Sickle cell disease*
Systemic lupus erythematosus
Eales' disease
Multiple sclerosis
Distal large artery occlusion
Takayasu's disease
Carotid artery obstruction
Coats' disease
Tumors
Retinal detachment
*Most frequently associated with retinal neovascularization

Table 1. Diseases associated with retinal neovascularization

Diseases Associated With Iris Neovascularization	
Vascular disorders	
Central retinal vein occlusion*	Central retinal artery occlusion
Branch retinal vein occlusion	Carotid occlusive disease
Takayasu's disease	Giant cell arteritis
Cartotid artery ligation	Carotid-cavernous fistula
Leber ciliary aneurysms	Retinopathy of prematurity
Sturge-Weber disease with choroidal hemangioma	
Ocular diseases	
Neovascular glaucoma*	Uveitis
Endophthalmitis	Vogt-Koyanagi syndrome
Retinal detachment	Persistent hyperplastic vitreous
Coats' disease	Eales' disease
Pseudoexfoliation of the lens capsule	
Sympathetic ophthalmia	Surgery and radiation therapy
Retinal detachment surgery	Vitrectomy
Laser coreoplasty	Cataract extraction
Radiation Trauma	
Systemic diseases	
Diabetes mellitus*	Norrie's disease
Sickle cell disease	Neurofibromatosis
Lupus erythematosus	Marfan's syndrome
Neoplastic diseases	
Retinoblastoma*	Melanoma of the choroid
Melanoma of the iris	Metastatic carcinoma
Reticulum cell sarcoma of ciliary body	

*Most frequently associated with iris neovascularization

Table 2. Diseases Associated With Iris Neovascularization

3. Prevalence and incidence

Overall incidence and prevalence of NVG has not been accurately reported, a retrospective study has shown a prevalence rate of 3.9%. The most common conditions associated with NVG are central retinal vein occlusion (CRVO), proliferative diabetic retinopathy (PDR), and other conditions such as ocular ischemic syndrome and tumors. Approximately 36% of NVG occurs after CRVO, 32% with PDR, and 13% occurs after carotid artery obstruction. Given that the underlying etiology of developing NVG is some form of retinal ischemia, it is more prevalent in elderly patients who have cardiovascular risk factors such as hypertension and diabetes, and may be more aggressive in those with obstructive sleep apnea syndrome (Shiba et al. 2009 and Shiba et al. 2011).

4. Physiopathology

Salus first observed abnormal vessels in the iris in 1928, calling the condition rubeosis iridis. Neovascularization of the iris (INV) is often followed by NVG, with its associated blindness and pain. (Laatikainen, 1979). The most common conditions that develop NVG as a complication of the disease are Diabetic Retinopathy (DR) and Central Retinal Vein Occlusion (CRVO), both having retinal hypoxia and ischemia as main contributory factor. (Al-Shamsi HN, Dueker DK, et, al. 2009)

Retinal hypoxia-ischemia increases the production of multiple factors: Vascular endothelial grow factor, nitric oxide, inflammatory cytokines, free radicals and accumulation of intracellular glutamate. (Charanjit Kaur et, al. 2008). The mechanism for reaching the critical level of retinal hypoxia-ischemia is different between DR and CRVO, because the first may need years to reach the level of VEGF that can develop INV and NVG, but CRVO could reach that level in only a few weeks.

4.1. Physiopathology of central retinal vein occlusion

Green made the most relevant histopathology study, in our opinion, in 1981. This study showed the natural history and characteristic evolution of thrombi in CRVO. First there is adherence of the thrombus to an area of the vein wall without its endothelium.

Inflammatory cell infiltration becomes prominent as a secondary factor. In early thrombosis, neutrophils may be seen clinging to the wall of the vein. After several weeks, a variable degree of lymphocyte infiltration was present in almost half of their cases. The infiltrate was seen in three places: around the vein (periphlebitis), in the wall of the vein (phlebitis) and/or in the occluded area. Endothelial-cell proliferation is an integral part of the process of organization and recanalization of the thrombus, and it occurs after several days.

In some of the eyes with an interval of a year or more between CRVO and the histologic study, a thick-walled vein with a single channel was present. They believe that these cases represent an old thrombus that now has a single or a main channel of recanalization. (Green, et al.1981)

Rubeosis iridis and NVG had a high prevalence in Green's study, reaching 82.8%. Other authors had previously described the high incidence of rubeosis iridis in CRVO, associated with clinical risk factors such as visual acuity less than 6/60 (20/200), more than 10 cotton-wool spots and/or severe retinal oedema seen by ophthalmoscopy. Some fluorescein angiography findings were also described, such as: severe capillary occlusion, prolonged arterio-venous transit time (over 20 seconds), posterior pole or peripheral severe large or small diameter vessel leakage. (Stephen H. Sinclair, Evangelos S. Gragoudas,1979). All these features are signs of hypoxia-ischemia and enhance the production of multiple vascular growth factors, the most important being vascular endothelial growth factor (VEGF).

4.2. Physiopathology of diabetic retinopathy

DR is widely regarded as a microvascular complication of diabetes. Clinically, DR can be classified into non-proliferative DR (NPDR) and proliferative DR (PDR) (Cheung et al., 2010. Remya Robinson, Veluchamy A. Et, al. 2012). In contrast to CRVO, the establishment of hypoxia-ischemia is slow. The transition between subsequent events caused by retinal hypoxia-ischemia in DR is reflected in the clinical classification. The most important factor that causes almost all vascular complications in diabetes mellitus is chronic hyperglycemia, although chronic hypoxia-reperfusion events may play an important role (Shiba et al. 2011).

The pathogenesis of the development of DR is complex and the exact mechanisms by which hyperglycemia initiates the vascular or neuronal alterations in DR have not been completely determined (Curtis et al., 2009; Villarroel et al., 2010; Remya Robinson, Veluchamy A. Et, al. 2012). Chronic hyperglycemia thickens the endothelial basement membrane of the capillaries and produces endothelial damage. Damaged endothelium can't be replaced properly because of perycite disfunction. Pericytes provide vascular stability and control endothelial proliferation, they are essential for the maturation of the developing vasculature.(Hans-Peter Hammes et, al. 2002).

Cellular damage could be caused by several mechanisms such as increased flux through the polyol pathway, production of advanced glycation end-products, increased oxidative stress and activation of the protein kinase C pathway, but many of these potential mechanisms remain as hypotheses. Chronic inflammatory response and the expression of vasoactive factors and cytokines may also play an important role in the pathogenesis of DR. (Remya Robinson, Veluchamy A. Et, al. 2012) In both CRVO and DR a hypoxic-ischemic retinal environment enhances the production of vascular proliferation factors, such as VEGF, in a dose-dependent manner, and the resultant rubeosis iridis is related to the degree of retinopathy, especially in proliferative diabetic retinopathy. (Francesco Bandello, Rosario Brancato, et, al. 1994)

4.3. Vascular Endothelial Growth Factor (VEGF)

One of the most important molecules involved in the pathogenesis of NVG is VEGF. This molecule is an endothelial cell specific angiogenic and vasopermeable factor (Lloyd Paul Aiello, Robert L Avery, et, al. 1994) and a molecule of convergence of various physiopathological mechanisms in both diseases.

VEGF incorporates five ligands (A, B, C, D & Placenta Growth Factor) that bind to three receptor tyrosine kinases (VEGFR-1 to 3). The founding member and the most characterized member is VEGF-A, for its angiogenic and permeability effects. VEGF-A binds to VEGFR-1 and 2, which may explain the properties of each regarding vascular permeability, angiogenesis, and survival. (Will Whitmire, Mohammed MH Al-Gayyar, et, al. 2011)

In the retina, VEGF-A is produced by retinal pigment epithelium (RPE), endothelial cells, pericytes, astrocytes, Muller cells, amacrine, and ganglion cells. (Will Whitmire, Mohammed MH Al-Gayyar, et, al. 2011).

There is a high level of VEGF in the anterior chamber of patients with ischemic CRVO and PDR. A close temporal correlation between aqueous VEGF levels and the degree of iris neovascularization has been demonstrated. (Sohan Singh Hayreh. 2007. Ciro Costagliola, Ugo Cipollone, et, al. 2008)

VEGF enhances the development of new abnormal vessels in the iris (INV) and the associated growth of fibrovascular tissue causes the formation of anterior synechiae and angle closure, which mechanically blocks aqueous humour outflow through the trabecular meshwork and increases intraocular pressure. (Ciro Costagliola, Ugo Cipollone, et, al. 2008)

A histopathological staging of eyes with neovascular glaucoma, according to the formation and extension of fibrovascular tissue in the anterior chamber angle and on the iris surface, has divided the condition into four stages. (Table 3, Figure 1)(Nomura T, Furukawa H, et, al. 1976).

Stage	Characteristics
1	Fibrovascular tissue occurs in the trabecular meshwork. Angle is open.
2	Fibrovascular tissue extends from the trabecular meshwork into the anterior chamber: peripheral anterior synechiae develop because of shrinkage of the fibrovascular tissue within the angle.
3	Fibrovascular tissue spreads on the anterior surface of the iris.
4	A single layer of endothelial cells develops on the surface of the fibrovascular membrane overlying the iris.

Table 3. Histopathological staging of neovascular glaucoma. (Nomura T, Furukawa H, et, al. 1976).

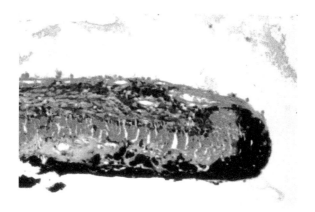

Figure 1. Fibrovascular tissue spreads on the anterior surface of the iris. The tissue pulls the posterior epithelial pigment of the iris over the pupil, causing ectropion uveae. Photography from Pathology Service, Asociación Para Evitar la Ceguera en México.

4.4. Physiopathology of optic nerve damage

VEGF, the main protein in the pathogenesis of NVG, plays a nonvascular and neuroprotective role in adult normal retinas. VEGF-A neutralization can cause neuroretinal cell apoptosis and loss of retinal function without affecting the normal vasculature of the retina. Treatment with VEGF-B protects retinal ganglion cells (RGC) in various models of neurotoxicity. This neuroprotective effect of VEGF-B was attributed to inhibition of pro-apoptotic proteins like p53 and caspases. The detrimental effects in environments with excessive VEGF-A, as happens in PDR, might be explained by excessive levels of peroxynitrite that can inhibit the VEGF-mediated survival signal via tyrosine nitration and subsequent inhibition of key survival proteins in retinal cells. (Will Whitmire, Mohammed MH Al-Gayyar, et, al. 2011).

Ischemia of the optic nerve head is the main reason of optic nerve damage in NVG. As the IOP rises the perfusion pressure decreases, worsening the ischemic condition of the optic nerve and retinal ganglion cells. (Ciro Costagliola, Ugo Cipollone, et, al. 2008).

5. Clinical manifestations and classifications

NVG could be underestimated in early stages of the disease, because there are very few signs that may be easily missed in a routine ophthalmologic exam. It's very important to identify patients who are at risk of developing NVG, specially those that have PDR or ischemic CRVO.

5.1. Early manifestations of neovascular glaucoma

INV could be seen like fine vessels at the pupillary margin in early stages, in fact INV starts in most cases at this level (Figure 2). In a small number of patients, neovascularization could start at the angle, making gonioscopy with an undilated pupil mandatory to all patients at risk of NVG. Careful gonioscopy is essential to detect early angle NV and early anterior synechiae. Other early signs often seen in NVG are flare, and sometimes a few cells, which may erroneously be diagnosed as a sign of uveitis.(Will Whitmire, Mohammed MH Al-Gayyar, et, al. 2011).

5.2. Late manifestations of neovascular glaucoma

Late manifestations of NVG appear when the disease is well established and the IOP is elevated. These include mid-peripheral neovascularization of the iris (Figure 3), neovascularization of the trabecular meshwork when the angle is still open, fibrovascular membrane over the iris and angle, peripheral anterior synechiaes, progressive angle closure and ectropion uvea.

5.3. Fluorescein iris angiogram classification

Fluorescein iris angiogram could help differentiate normal iris vessels from INV. The vascular abnormalities revealed by fluorescein angiography of the iris are: dilated leaking vessels around the pupil, irregular or slow filling of the radial arteries, superficial arborizing neovascularization, usually starting in the angle; and dilatation and leakage of the radial vessels, particularly the arteries. (Leila Laatikainen, 1979). On the basis of angiographic findings, diabetic iridopathy was divided in 4 grades (Table 4).

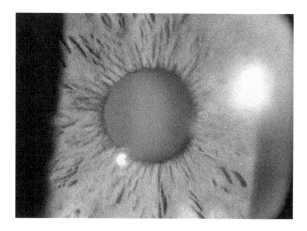

Figure 2. Early rubeosis at the pupillary margin. Photography from the Glaucoma Service, Asociación Para Evitar la Ceguera en México.

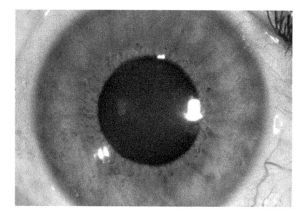

Figure 3. Late rubeosis with mid-peripheral neovascularization of the iris. Photography from the Glaucoma Service, Asociación Para Evitar la Ceguera en México.

Grade	Findings
1	Peripupillary vessel dilatations, Dilated leaking capillaries around the pupil, Irregularities in the filling of radial vessels
2	Early neovascularization of the angle (gonioscopy) Arborizing superficial, early, new vessels Filling of vessels in the early arterial phase and leakage of fluorescein
3	Prominent rubeosis with or without NVG Prominent arborizing new vessels grown out of the angle, covering a larger iris surface Filling of new vessels in early arterial phase Generalized marked leakage
4	Florid rubeosis Complete angle closure New vessels covering the entire iris surface Eversion of the pigmented border of the pupil

Table 4. Classification of rubeosis iridis in diabetic eye disease. (Leila Laatikainen, 1979).

In preproliferative and proliferative DR, iris fluorescein angiogram detection of iris neovessels has a reported sensitivity of 56% and a specificity of 100%. (Francesco Bandello, Rosario Brancato. 1994).

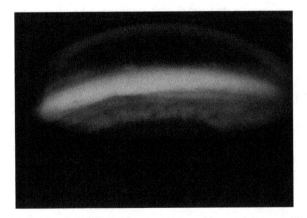

Figure 4. Neovascularization of the trabecular meshwork and anterior peripheral synechiae. Photography from the Glaucoma Service, Asociación Para Evitar la Ceguera en México.

5.4. Clinical classifications

A clinical grading system was also proposed in order to guide pan-retinal photocoagulation therapy, and to select patients who will respond well to the treatment. (Table 5) (Teich SA,

Walsh JB, 1981). This classification is no longer used in our glaucoma service, because treatment has changed with the use of antiangiogenic drugs.

Grade	
0	Absence of iris neovascularization
1	Neovascularization of the pupillary zone less than 2 quadrants
2	Neovascularization of the pupillary zone more than 2 quadrants
3	Neovascularization of the pupillary zone more than 2 quadrants + ectropion uvea or less than 2 quadrants at iris ciliary zone
4	Ectropion uvea and more than 3 quadrants of neovascularization at the iris ciliary zone

Table 5. Clinical grading system of Iris Neovascularization. (Teich SA, Walsh JB, 1981).

In order to differentiate patients for specific treatments, we classify NVG patients in three stages, depending on the characteristics of the angle, the iris and IOP, since the advent of anti-angiogenics and their rapid onset of action has made the amount of iris neovascularization irrelevant in the absence of angle closure. (Castaneda-Díez, García-Aguirre, 2010.)

Grade	Characteristics
1	Early Iris or angle neovascularization with open angle and normal IOP
2	Clinically evident Iris or angle neovascularization with open angle and IOP between 20 and 30 mmHg.
3	Prominent iris and/or angle neovascularization with angle closure, ectropion uvea and IOP over 30 mmHg.

Table 6. Clinical classification of Neovascular Glaucoma. (Castaneda-Díez, García-Aguirre, 2010.)

6. Medical and surgical treatment of neovascular glaucoma

The management of neovascular glaucoma is summarized in figure 5, and depends on whether the angle is open or closed, and whether media are clear or not in order to correctly visualize the retina. Management can be divided in:

Measures to decrease the amount of VEGF produced by the retina, or its effects: Pan-retinal photocoagulation, antiangiogenic drugs and/or pars-plana vitrectomy.

Measures to control intraocular pressure: Medications to reduce intraocular pressure and/or filtering procedures.

6.1. Pan-retinal photocoagulation

Neovascular glaucoma is best treated with prevention. Since retinal ischemia (and VEGF production) is the main predisposing factor for the development of rubeosis iridis, angle neovascularization and NVG, laser photocoagulation to the areas of retinal ischemia continues to be one of the mainstays of treatment, and should be performed promptly in patients with NVG that have media clear enough for the treatment to be delivered.

The rationale behind pan-retinal photocoagulation (PRP) is to preserve central vision, if possible, by sacrificing peripheral vision. Retinal ablation is thought to reduce the metabolic needs of the hypoxic retina by reducing the total amount of functional retina, so remaining retinal circulation is sufficient to prevent further production of vessel growth factors by the non-ablated retinal tissue.

For the treatment to be applied correctly, a fluorescein angiogram is necessary, in order to determine the presence of areas of retinal non-perfusion and retinal neovascularization. Treatment is applied under pharmacologic mydriasis, using a wide-field contact lens (such as the Super-Quad or Mainster lenses). The parameters for retinal photocoagulation used in the ETDRS are preferred (ETDRS, 1987: A spot diameter of 500 μm, 100 msec duration and enough power to produce a gray-whitish burn on the retina, with a separation between spots of 250 μm), and the whole treatment is delivered in one session, if possible, in order to ablate the largest area of retina possible.

If there are concerns regarding possible complications of an excessive photocoagulation, such as serous retinal detachment or choroidal detachment, reduced fluence parameters may be used (spot diameter of 500 μm, 20 msec duration and power enough to produce a gray-whitish burn on the retina), which have proven to be effective, (Muqit MM, 2011) and to cause less discomfort to the patient (Alvarez-Verduzco O, Garcia-Aguirre G, 2010). These reduced fluence parameters may be used with the Pattern Scan Laser (PaScaL photocoagulator, OptiMedica) (Velez-Montoya R, Guerrero-Naranjo JL, 2010), or with a standard 532 nm laser (Alvarez-Verduzco O, Garcia-Aguirre G, 2010).

PRP has proven to be effective for the prevention of neovascular glaucoma secondary to diabetic retinopathy (The Diabetic Retinopathy Study Research Group, 1976) and central retinal vein occlusion, (Central Vein Occlusion Study Group, 1996) which are the most frequent causal entities. Some concerns have been raised, however, regarding the efficacy of this treatment in central retinal vein occlusion (Hayreh SS, 2007).

The timing of PRP is critical, regarding final visual acuity and NVG prevention. It takes about 4 weeks for PRP to show regression of anterior segment neovascularization (ASNV), and this is thought to depend on the pre-existing levels of vitreous growth factors, mainly vascular endothelial growth factor (VEGF). Once PRP stops the hypoxic retina from producing additional growth factors, existing VEGF and other factors remain in the vitreous for a period during which additional vessel growth may still occur under their influence.

To further complicate matters, a PRP treatment may need 2 or 3 sessions in order to be complete (2000 to 2500 shots), and these sessions are frequently done 2 to 4 weeks apart to avoid excessive inflammation. The period between sessions before a full-treatment has been given is also a period during which further VEGF production may be taking place, especially in the most hypoxic retinas.

6.2. Antiangiogenic drugs

As stated above, VEGF is the main molecule responsible for the development of neovascularization, and therefore neovascular glaucoma. Pan-retinal photocoagulation is very effective for long-term suppression of VEGF, but the decline of such levels tends to take place gradually after treatment, which in theory could leave a time window for the disease to progress. Besides, the need of clear media for PRP treatment of most, if not all, the hypoxic retina may also increase the time before those VEGF levels begin to decrease. To address this problem, anti-VEGF drugs have proven to be of great value.

Since their appearance, both bevacizumab and later ranibizumab (Avastin and Lucentis, Genentech-Roche, South San Francisco, CA) have been used as adjuvants for the treatment of neovascular glaucoma. Injection of a single dose in most cases results in brisk disappearance of iris and/or angle neovascularization (Kahook MY, 2006).

The administration of bevacizumab has been shown to dramatically reduce VEGF levels in the aqueous humor after intracameral injection (Sasamoto Y, 2012) and to reduce edema, fibrin deposition, inflammation and vascular congestion in trabecular meshwork specimens obtained during trabeculectomy performed after intravitreal injection.(Yoshida N, 2011) Several studies have found intravitreal bevacizumab to be of great value as an adjunct to the treatment of neovascular glaucoma of diverse etiologies, causing prompt regression of anterior segment neovascularization (ASNV), and better control of intraocular pressure.(Ehlers JP, 2008. Wakabayashi T, 2008. Yazdani S, 2009. Beutel J. 2010) Good results have also been obtained with ranibizumab (Caujolle JP, 2012), although there are fewer studies in the literature describing the use of this drug.

These agents have also been used for reducing fibrosis in failed filtering blebs (Kahook MY, 2006b) and even for wound modulation in primary trabeculectomies (Horsley et al, 2010) and Ahmed valve implants (Rojo-Arnao, Albis-Donado et al, 2011). A similar trend has been observed with Ranibizumab, a drug designed for intraocular delivery, with an expanding range of on- and off-label indications (Kumar et al, 2012, Mota et al. 2012, Desai et al. 2012, Auila JS, 2012), especially since a potentially deleterious accumulation of Bevacizumab in retinal pigment epithelial cells (Deissler at al. 2012) and approval of Ranibizumab in Europe (and more recently by the FDA) for diabetic macular edema have recently further increased its use despite a greater cost per dose.

As with any procedure, there are complications that have been reported with the use of anti-VEGF drugs. Most of the adverse effects are the ones expected with any intraocular injection, such as subconjunctival hemorrhage, lens damage, or endophthalmitis (Gordon-Angelozzi M, 2009). Other complications, however, are not related to the procedure but to the effect of the drug itself, such as a decrease in the electroretinogram response (Wittström E, 2012), central retinal artery occlusion in eyes with ocular ischemic syndrome (Higashide T, 2012), abrupt angle closure (Canut MI, 2011), or induction of tractional retinal detachment in eyes with abundant retinal neovascular proliferations (Torres-Soriano M, 2009. Arevalo JF, 2008), and should therefore be used with caution in patients at risk.

When anti-angiogenics are used before angle-closure has happened, ASNV regression will prevent IOP elevation, it may revert IOP elevation associated with angle neovessels or at least make it amenable to be medically controlled, and, subsequently, it can also prevent angle-closure and a more aggressive IOP elevation. During this period the media may clear enough for PRP to be completed or initiated.

6.3. Medical management of glaucoma

Once IOP is elevated in NVG cases medical therapy with aqueous production suppressors should be initiated. Topical beta-blockers, topical and oral carbonic anhydrase inhibitors and alpha-2-adrenergic agonists are used, whereas prostaglandin analogues, should not be used because they increase inflammation and may not even lower IOP, unless ASNV has regressed and has a low chance of reappearing, although the exact IOP lowering and safety profile in these patients is still in controversy.

Topical corticosteroids are used concurrently to treat associated inflammation, and may actually help to prevent further angle closure during the initial phase. Atropine may also be used for its cycloplegic effect, but in addition to increasing uveoscleral outflow and maybe lower IOP, it may also help prevent miotic pupillary block, stabilize the blood-aqueous barrier and facilitate posterior segment visualization and treatment. Pilocarpine and other anticholinergic agents are contra-indicated, as they increase inflammation, cause miosis, worsen synechial angle closure and decrease uveoscleral outflow.

In most cases of NVG in closed angle-phases, medical therapy may not be enough to control IOP and prevent visual loss. (Kurt Spiteri Cornish. 2011). If angle-closure has already happened an Ahmed valve-implant is recommended. It may also be needed for around 15% of open-angle phase NVG that remain with elevated IOP, despite anti-angiogenic therapy and adequate PRP. The immediate effect of previously administered intra-vitreous anti-angiogenics during surgery is a reduced tendency for bleeding at the time of tube insertion. On the long term a tendency for better IOP control has been reported (Desai et al. 2012).

6.4. Surgical management of neovascular glaucoma

6.4.1. Tube-shunt surgery

Glaucoma implants have made it possible to save many eyes with NVG from becoming blind, painful eyes. They have also made it possible to preserve useful vision, specially when IOP can be controlled from the day surgery is performed. Using non-valved implants (such as Barveldt or Molteno setons) requires the use of hypotony prevention strategies that have included a two-stage operation, tying off the tube with an absorbable suture or the use of a suture threaded inside the tube.

The idea is to let fibrous tissue grow around the implant, forming a semi-permeable barrier that will eventually absorb excess aqueous. Depending on the chosen strategy, the opening of the implant can be programmed for a couple of weeks in the future for the removable suture or the second stage procedure, or it may happen on its own 3 to 6 weeks later for the absorbable suture.

Since many eyes might still have elevated IOP during this period, damage to the optic nerve may become so advanced as to make the eye legally or even fully blind. A metanalysis comparing restrictive and non-restrictive implants has shown that the mean rate of decrease in visual acuity tends to be lower for the Ahmed valve (19 to 24%) as compared to the other devices (27 to 33%, Hong et al. 2005, Albis-Donado 2009). IOP control from day one and subsequent better visual results have made the Ahmed valve the implant of choice in our hospital for NVG.

Our simpler surgical technique, without the use of a scleral graft patch, has been routinely used for the past 19 years and has been described elsewhere (Gil-Carrasco et al.1998, Albis-Donado, 2006, Albis-Donado et al. 2010). In brief, a fornix-based conjunctival flap is made in the designated quadrant, and then the valve is primed with BSS and fixated 8 to 10 mm behind the limbus with 7-0 silk. A scleral tunnel initiated 3-4 mm from the limbus is constructed using a 22 or 23 G needle, bent as a "Z" to avoid obstruction from the eyelids, brow or lid speculum.

The needle is passed bevel-up under the episclera, in a tangential direction; at the limbus the direction is abruptly changed to make the tunnel parallel to the iris, attempting to enter through the trabecular meshwork. The tube is then trimmed to create a 30-45º bevel and inserted through the tunnel into the anterior chamber, leaving the tip at least 2 mm from the limbus. The conjunctiva is closed using the same 7-0 silk in cooperating adults. Post-operative regimen includes steroid drops in a reducing dose for 3 months, antibiotic drops for 2 weeks, and a cycloplegic for the first month.

The most common complications after an Ahmed valve implant in NVG are hyphema (up to 45% without bevacizumab, and reduced to about 8% with an injection 1 day before the implant), and flat anterior chamber (around 32%, especially in phakic eyes, Albis-Donado et al, 2012).

In the long term the most common complication is elevation of IOP during the so termed hypertensive phase, but that might become permanent, both are thought to occur due to fibrosis around the plate. A tendency for lower rates of IOP elevation with the use of antiangiogenic drugs has been reported (Ehlers JP, 2008. Wakabayashi T, 2008. Yazdani S, 2009. Beutel J. 2010, Rojo-Arnao et al, 2011, Caujolle JP, 2012).

Removal of the fibrous tissue around the implant, adjuvant aqueous suppressants and massage might also be of value for the long-term of IOP control.

6.4.2. Pars plana vitrectomy

A significant proportion of eyes with neovascular glaucoma have significant media opacities that preclude adequate panretinal photocoagulation. In such cases, vitreoretinal surgery plays an important role in its management, since it allows to clear the media opacities, to repair the damaged posterior segment and/or to deliver laser treatment via endophotocoagulation probes. For this reason, several studies have been conducted to explore the usefulness of posterior segment procedures for the treatment of neovascular glaucoma, most of the time performed in conjunction with filtering surgery.

One of the earliest studies was published in 1982 by Sinclair et al, who performed pars plana vitrectomy and lensectomy, and an sclerectomy in 14 eyes with neovascular glaucoma, with poor results. After six months, 64% of eyes had maintained or improved visual acuity, 7% had decreased visual acuity, and 28% lost light perception. This procedure had several complications, including fibrinous vitritis (71%), suprachoroidal hemorrhage (14%), endophthalmitis (7%), retinal detachment (7%) and phthisis bulbi (14%).

Several years later, in 1991, Lloyd et al reported the results of a study in which pars plana vitrectomy and a pars plana Molteno implant were performed in 10 eyes, achieving control of intraocular pressure (21 mmHg or less) in 6 of them. However, three eyes developed vitreous hemorrhage, three developed retinal detachment and two lost light perception.

In 1993, Gandham et al published a study of 20 eyes with glaucoma of difficult management (8 out of which had neovascular glaucoma), that underwent pars plana vitrectomy, and placement of a Molteno or Schocket implant. In six out of the eight eyes (75%), an intraocular pressure of 22 mmHg or less was achieved.

In 1995, Luttrull and Avery reported 22 eyes in which pars plana vitrectomy and a pars plana Molteno implant placement were performed. As an additional procedure, either a ligature of the implant tube with absorbable suture or perfluropropane gas tamponade were performed, in order to avoid postoperative hypotony. With this procedure, an intraocular pressure of 21 mmHg or less was achieved in all eyes, and stabilization or improvement of visual acuity was achieved in 86% of eyes. Among the postoperative complications, retinal detachement was observed in two eyes, and loss of light perception in one eye.

More recently, Faghihi et al in 2007 published their experience in 18 eyes with neovascular glaucoma that underwent pars plana vitrectomy and pars plana Ahmed valve implant. An intraocular pressure of 21 or less was achieved in 13 eyes (72.2%). Light perception was lost in two eyes and two evolved to phthisis bulbi.

In these four studies, the justification to introduce the tube through the pars plana into the vitreous cavity instead of the anterior chamber was to avoid complications such as hyphema or blockage of the tube by a fibrovascular membrane.

6.4.3. Cycloablation

The main goal in the struggle with neovascular glaucoma in blind eyes is to control intraocular pressure (IOP) and pain. (A Janićijević-Petrović M, 2012). In one prospective study the average value of IOP and eyeball pain intensity was significantly lower after cyclocryocoagulation. Cyclocryocoagulation could be a good method in the treatment of uncontrolled elevated IOP and pain of progressive NVG resistant to medical and surgical treatment, but does not have any effect on the improvement of sight in these patients. (Kovacić Z, Ivanisević M, 2004)

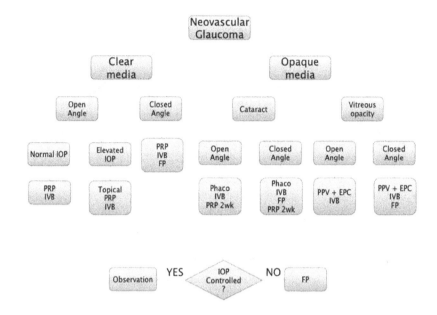

Figure 5. Management of Neovascular Glaucoma. IOP: Intraocular pressure; PRP: Panretinal photocoagulation; IVB: Intravitreal bevacizumab; Topical IOP lowering drugs; FP: Filtering procedure (Ahmed valve); PRP 2wk: Panretinal photocoagulation 2 weeks after the procedure PPV+EPC: Pars plana vitrectomy and endophotocoagulation.

7. Conclusions

The physiopathology of NVG involves various biochemical and biological mechanisms that result in the presence of abnormal vessels that lead to the clinical forms of the disease. This natural history can be modified and steered into a more appropriate and less devastating behavior, depending on the sagacity of the physician and the commitment that the patient has to his/her own condition.

One fundamental aspect of NVG management is the treatment of the underlying condition that caused it. Uncontrolled diabetes, systemic hypertension, vascular diseases, and even primary open angle glaucoma are all modifiable factors that may reduce the incidence of NVG. Periodic ophthalmology visits for patients at risk should be part of their primary care, especially since the prevalence of these systemic conditions seems to be on the rise.

What used to be a condition that was a synonym for irreversible, painful blindness is now expected to be controllable to a degree compatible with useful vision, but through a challenging course of treatment.

Three strategies for preserving vision have increasingly improved the visual prognosis in NVG patients. First was the advent of Panretinal Photocoagulation, when done on time prevented or treated the worst cases of NVG.

The second strategy, and probably the most pivotal turning point, was the arrival of Ahmed valves, permitting control of IOP from day 1, and, in conjunction with PRP, preserving useful vision for the first time without the frequent failures of trabeculectomies. In our initial series (Gil-Carrasco et al. 1997) 137 NVG eyes had a preoperative IOP of 36.7 (SD 11.2) and it lowered to 13.7 (SD 3.4), around 80% were successful at 12 months. Shunt devices have gained in popularity for the management of NVG.

The third and newest strategy has been the incorporation of anti-angiogenic agents from the beginning of this century. Our group performed a prospective study on the use of 2.5 mg of intravitreal Bevacizumab plus PRP in 36 patients who had rubeosis iridis (group A), NVG in open-angle phase (Group B) or NVG with at least 180 degrees of angle closure (Group C).

At 1 week all eyes had regression of all visible anterior segment neovascularization. Additionally in group B, survival of adequate IOP control using only topical medications, without progressing to closed-angle phase, was 90% at 3 months, 81% at 6 months, and 70.9% at 9, 12 and 18 months. All eyes in group C had an Ahmed valve implant (AVI) within 96 hours of the intravitreal injection without serious complications, observing only scant intraoperative bleeding in one eye and a 1 mm hyphema in 2 other eyes on the first postoperative day. Kaplan-Meier analysis of group C showed survival of post-AVI IOP control, without further interventions, of 100% at 6 months, 85.7% at 9,12 and 18 months of follow-up. Survival rate for neovessel-free anterior segment was 75%, 57.7% and 62.5% at 18 months in groups A, B and C, respectively.

We concluded that Preoperative intravitreal Bevacizumab has an important role as an adjuvant to pan-retinal photocoagulation in neovessels regression, controlling IOP and avoiding angle-closure in open-angle NVG, and for reducing bleeding after Ahmed Valve implantation.

A recent review of 912 Ahmed valve implants without a patch, followed for up to 16 years at our hospital found a 49% success rate for avoiding blindness and maintaining IOP under 21 mmHg. There were 363 NVG cases (39.8%), by far the most frequent indication for Ahmed valve implants and most of them associated with diabetic retinopathy (Gil-Carrasco et al. 2012).

The combination of Ahmed valve implants, anti-angiogenics and full PRP, plus topical anti-glaucoma medications as needed, has become the spearhead in the management of neovascular glaucoma at our institution. New surgical approaches for NVG and a better understanding of the disease offer an encouraging perspective for the visual prognosis of these patients.

Author details

Cynthia Esponda-Lammoglia, Rafael Castaneda-Díez, Gerardo García-Aguirre, Oscar Albis-Donado and Jesús Jiménez-Román

Asociación para Evitar la Ceguera en México, Mexico City, Mexico

References

[1] Al-Shamsi HN, Dueker DK, Nowilaty SR, Al-Shahwan SA.Middle East Afr J Oph-thalmol. Neovascular glaucoma at king khaled eye specialist hospital - etiologic con-siderations.2009 Jan;16(1):15-9.

[2] Albert Daniel M. et al. Albert and Jakobiec`s Principles and Practice of Ophthalmolo-gy. Chapter 213. Neovascular Glaucoma

[3] Albis-Donado O. Chapter 6:The Ahmed Valve. In Shaarawy T. and Mermoud A. (eds). Atlas of Glaucoma Surgery, Jaypee Brothers, New Delhi, India, 2006: 58-76.

[4] Albis-Donado O. Chapter 104 – "Drainage Implants – Results", in "Glaucoma – First Edition", Shaarawy, Sherwood, Hitchings, and Crowston (eds) – Elsevier-Saunders, 2009.

[5] Albis-Donado O, Gil-Carrasco F, Romero Quijada R, Thomas R. Evaluation of ahmed glaucoma valve implantation through a needle-generated scleral tunnel in Mexican children with glaucoma. Indian J Ophthalmol 2010;58:365-73.

[6] Albis-Donado O., Mayorquín-Ruiz M., Soto-Ortiz K., Gil-Carrasco F. "Factores de riesgo para cámara plana en válvulas de Ahmed para Glaucoma Neovascular en la era pre-Bevacizumab", Revista Mexicana de Oftalmología, Vol. 86. Num. 01. Enero - Marzo 2012.

[7] A Janićijević-Petrović M, Sarenac T, Petrović M, Vulović D, Janićijević K. Cyclocryo-therapy in neovascular glaucoma treatment. Med Glas Ljek komore Zenicko-doboj kantona. 2012 Feb;9(1):106-8.

[8] Alvarez-Verduzco O, Garcia-Aguirre G, Lopez-Ramos Mde L, Vera-Rodriguez S, Guerrero-Naranjo JL, Morales-Canton V. Reduction of fluence to decrease pain dur-ing panretinal photocoagulation in diabetic patients. Ophthalmic Surg Lasers Imag-ing. 2010;4:432-6.

[9] Arevalo JF, Maia M, Flynn HW Jr, et al. Tractional retinal detachment following in-travitreal bevacizumab (Avastin) in patients with severe proliferative diabetic retin-opathy. Br J Ophthalmol 2008;92:213-216.

[10] Aujla JS. Replacing ranibizumab with bevacizumab on the Pharmaceutical Benefits Scheme: where does the current evidence leave us? Clin Exp Optom. 2012 May 24

[11] Beutel J, Peters S, Lüke M, Aisenbrey S, Szurman P, Spitzer MS, Yoeruek E; Bevacizu-mab Study Group, Grisanti S. Bevacizumab as adjuvant for neovascular glaucoma. Acta Ophthalmol. 2010;88:103-9.

[12] Brown GC, Magargal LE, Schachat A, Shah J. Neovascular Glaucoma. Etiologic con-siderations. Ophthalmology 1984;91:315-320.

[13] Canut MI, Alvarez A, Nadal J, Abreu R, Abreu JA, Pulido JS. Anterior segment changes following intravitreal bevacizumab injection for treatment of neovascular glaucoma. Clin Ophthalmol 2011;5:715-9.

[14] Caujolle JP, Maschi C, Freton A, Pages G, Gastaud P. Treatment of neovascular glaucoma after proton therapy for uveal melanomas with ranibizumab injection: preliminary results. Ophthalmic Res 2012;47:57-60.

[15] Central Vein Occlusion Study Group. The CVOS Group M and N Reports. Ophthalmology 1996;103:353-354.

[16] Chan. Clement K MD, et al. SCORE Study Report # 11. Incidence of Neovascular Events in Eyes with Retinal Vein Occlusion. Ophthalmology 2011; 118: 1364-1372.

[17] Charanjit Kaur, Wallace S, Foulds, Eng-Ang Ling, Hypoxia-ischemia and retinal ganglion cell damage. Clinical Ophthalmology 2008:2(4) 879–889 879

[18] Cheung, N., Mitchell, P. and Wong, T. Y. (2010). Diabetic retinopathy. Lancet 376, 124- 136.

[19] Ciro Costagliola, Ugo Cipollone, Michele Rinaldi, Michele della Corte, Francesco Semeraro & Mario R. Romano. Intravitreal bevacizumab injection for neovascular glaucoma: a survey on 23 cases throughout 12-month follow-up. British Journal of Clinical Pharmacology. 2008 / 66:5 / 667673

[20] Clemens A.K. Lange, Panagiotis Stavrakas, Ulrich FO Luhmann, Don Julian de Silva, Robin R Ali, Zdenek J Gregor, James Bainbridge. Intraocular Oxygen Distribution in Advanced Proliferative Retinopathy. Am J Ophthalmol 2011; 152: 406-412.

[21] Curtis, T. M., Gardiner, T. A. and Stitt, A. W. (2009). Microvascular lesions of diabetic retinopathy: clues towards understanding pathogenesis. Eye 23, 1496-1508.

[22] Desai RU, Singh K, Lin AS. Intravitreal ranibizumab as an adjunct for ahmed valve surgery in open angle glaucoma: a pilot study. Clin Experiment Ophthalmol. 2012 Jun 19.

[23] Deissler HL, Deissler H, Lang GE. Actions of bevacizumab and ranibizumab on microvascular retinal endothelial cells: similarities and differences. Br J Ophthalmol. 2012 Jul;96(7):1023-8.

[24] Domínguez-Dueñas, F., Albis-Donado, O., Thomas, R., Monges-Ureña, L., García-Huerta, M., Gil-Carrasco, F. "Intravitreal Bevacizumab in rubeosis iridis and neovascular glaucoma: Prospective 18 months follow-up", 4th International Congress on Glaucoma Surgery, Geneva, Switzerland, April 2009.

[25] Early Treatment Diabetic Retinopathy Study Research Group: Treatment techniques and clinical guidelines for photocoagulation of diabetic macular edema. Early Treatment Diabetic Retinopathy Study Report Number 2. Ophthalmology 1987;94: 761-774

[26] Ehlers JP, Spirn MJ, Lam A, Sivalingam A, Samuel MA, Tasman W. Combination intravitreal bevacizumab/panretinal photocoagulation versus panretinal photocoagulation alone in the treatment of neovascular glaucoma. Retina. 2008;28:696-702.

[27] Faghihi H, Hajizadeh F, Mohammadi SF, et al. Pars plana Ahmed valve implant and vitrectomy in the management of neovascular glaucoma. Ophthalmic Surg Lasers Imaging 2007;38:292-300

[28] Francesco Bandello, Rosario Brancato, Rosangela Lattanzio, Marcello Galdini, Bruno Falcomata. Relation between iridopathy and retinopathy in diabetes. British Journal of Ophthalmology 1994; 78: 542-545.

[29] Gandham SB, Costa VP, Katz LJ, et al. Aqueous tube-shunt implantation and pars plana vitrectomy in eyes with refractory glaucoma. Am J Ophthalmol 1993;116:189-195.

[30] Gil Carrasco F, Paczka JA, Jiménez Román J, Gilbert Lucido ME, De los Ríos D, Sánchez Castellanos VE Experiencia clínica inicial con la válvula de Ahmed: reporte de 278 casos con glaucoma incontrolable. St Ophthal, 16:117-122, 1997 (Available online: http://www.oftalmo.com/studium/studium1997/stud97-2/b-02.htm)

[31] Gil-Carrasco F, Salinas-VanOrman E, Recillas-Gispert C, Paczka JA, Gilbert ME, Arellanes-Garcia L. Ahmed valve implant for uncontrolled uveitic glaucoma. Ocul Immunol Inflamm. 1998 Mar;6(1):27-37.

[32] Gil-Carrasco F., Albis-Donado O., Castañeda-Diez R., Turati-Acosta M., Garcia-Huerta M., Jimenez-Roman J. Long-term results in 912 Ahmed valves without graft patch in Mexico: 16 years of follow-up. 6th International Congress on Glaucoma Surgery, Glasgow, Scotland UK 2012.

[33] Gordon-Angelozzi M, Velez-Montoya R, Fromow-Guerra J, García-Aguirre G, Guerrero-Naranjo JL, Quiroz-Mercado H, Morales-Cantón V. Bevacizumab local complications. Ophthalmology 2009;116:2264.

[34] Hans-Peter Hammes et al, Pericytes and the Pathogenesis of Diabetic Retinopathy, Diabetes 51(10):3107-3112, 2002.

[35] Hayreh SS. Neovascular Glaucoma. Prog Ret Eye Res 2007;26:470-485.

[36] Hidehar Funatsu, MD, Hidetoshi Yamashita, MD, Hidekata Noma, MD, Tatsuya Mimura MD, tetsuji Yamashita and Sadao Hori Md. Increased Levels of Vascular Endothelial Growth Factor and Interleukin-6 in the Aqueous Humor of Diabetics with Macular Edema. Am J Ophthalmol 2002; 133: 70-77.

[37] Higashide T, Murotani E, Saito Y, Ohkubo S, Sugiyama K. Adverse events associated with intraocular injections of bevacizumab in eyes with neovascular glaucoma. Graefes Arch Clin Exp Ophthalmol 2012;250:603-10.

[38] Hong CH, Arosemena A, Zurakowski D, et al. Glaucoma drainage devices: a systematic literature review and current controversies. Surv Ophthalmol 2005; 50:48–60.

[39] Horsley MB, Kahook MY. Anti-VEGF therapy for glaucoma. Curr Opin Ophthalmol. 2010 Mar;21(2):112-7.

[40] Kahook MY, Schuman JS, Noecker RJ. Intravitreal bevacizumab in a patient with neovascular glaucoma. Ophthalmic Surg Lasers Imaging 2006;37:144-6.

[41] Kahook MY, Schuman JS, Noecker RJ. Needle bleb revision of encapsulated filtering bleb with bevacizumab. Ophthalmic Surg Lasers Imaging. 2006 Mar-Apr;37(2): 148-50.

[42] Ko-Hua Chen, Chih-Chiau Wu, Sayon Roy, Shui-Mei Lee, Jorn-Hon Liu. Increased Interleukin-6 in Aqueous Humor of Neovascular Glaucoma. Invest Ophthalmol Vis Sci. 1999; 40: 2627-2632.

[43] Kovacić Z, Ivanisević M, Rogosić V, Plavec A, Karelović D. Cyclocryocoagulation in treatment of neovascular glaucoma. Lijec Vjesn. 2004 Sep-Oct;126(9-10):240-2.

[44] Kumar B, Gupta SK, Saxena R, Srivastava S. Current trends in the pharmacotherapy of diabetic retinopathy. J Postgrad Med. 2012 Apr;58(2):132-9.

[45] Kurt Spiteri Cornish. Neovascular Glaucoma. Glaucoma – Current Clinical and Research Aspects. 2011. Kurt Spiteri Cornish (2011). Neovascular Glaucoma, Glaucoma - Current Clinical and Research Aspects, Pinakin Gunvant (Ed.), ISBN: 978-953-307-263-0, InTech.

[46] Lee, Patricia MD, Wang, Cindy. MD, Adamis P, Anthony. Ocular Neovascularization and the Eye. Survey of Ophthalmology.1998: 43;245-269.

[47] Leila Laatikainen, Development and classification of rubeosis iridis in diabetic eye disease. British Journal of Ophthalmology, 1979, 63, 150-156

[48] Lloyd MA, Heuer DK, Baerveldt G, et al. Combined Molteno implantation and pars plana vitrectomy for neovascular glaucoma. Ophthalmology 1991;98:1401-1405.

[49] Lloyd Paul Aiello, Robert L Avery, Paul G Arrigg, Bruce A Keyt, Henry D Jampel, Sabera T Shah, Louis R Pasquale, Hagen Thieme, Mami A. Iwamoto, John E Park, Hung V. Nguyen, M.S.,Lloyd M. Aiello, Napoleone Ferrara and George L. King. Vascular Endothelial Growth Factor in Ocular Fluid of Patients With diabetic Retinopathy and Other Retinal Disorders. N Engl J Med 1994;331:1480-7.

[50] Luttrull JK, Avery RL. Pars plana implant and vitrectomy for treatment of neovascular glaucoma. Retina 1995;15:379-387.

[51] Machintosh B. Rachel, Rogers. Sophie L, Lim. Lyndell, Ning. Cheung, Wang. Jie Jin, Mitchell. Paul, Kowalski. Jonathan. Natural History Of Central Retinal Vein Occlusion: An Evidence Based Systematic Review. Ophthalmology 2010; 117: 1113-1123.

[52] Mota A, Carneiro A, Breda J, Rosas V, Magalhães A, Silva R, Falcão-Reis F. Combina-
      tion of intravitreal ranibizumab and laser photocoagulation for aggressive posterior
      retinopathy of prematurity. Case Report Ophthalmol. 2012 Jan;3(1):136-41.

[53] Muqit MM, Marcellino GR, Henson DB, Young LB, Turner GS, Stanga PE. Pascal
      panretinal laser ablation and regression analysis in proliferative diabetic retinopathy:
      Manchester Pascal Study Report 4. Eye 2011;25(11):1447-56

[54] Nomura T, Furukawa H, Kurimoto S. Development and classification of neovascular
      glaucoma in diabetic eye disease: histopathological study. Acta Ophthalmol Soc J7pn
      1976;86: 166-75.

[55] Pe'er. Jacob MD, Folberg. Robert MD, Itin. Ahwa, Gnessin. Hadassah, Hemo. Itzhak
      MD, Keshet. Eli PhD. Vascular Endothelial Growth Factor Up regulation in Human
      Central Retinal Vein Occlusion. Ophthalmology 1998;105: 412-416.

[56] Castañeda-Díez R., García-Aguirre G. Vitrectomía en Pacientes Diabéticos con Glau-
      coma Neovascular, Highlights of vitreoretina, 2010

[57] Remya Robinson, Veluchamy A. Barathi,, Shyam S. Chaurasia, Tien Y. Wong and
      Timothy S. Ker. Update on animal models of diabetic retinopathy: from molecular
      approaches to mice and higher mammals.Disease Models & Mechanisms 5, 444-456
      (2012)

[58] Richard Green, MD, Chi Chao Chan, MD, CRVO: A prospective histopathologic
      study of 29 eyes in 28, Tr. Am. Ophth. Soc. vol. LXXIX,1981.

[59] Rojo-Arnao M, Albis-Donado OD, Lliteras-Cardin M, Kahook MY, Gil-Carrasco F.
      Adjunctive bevacizumab in patients undergoing Ahmed valve implantation: a pilot
      study. Ophthalmic Surg Lasers Imaging. 2011 Mar-Apr;42(2):132-7.

[60] Sasamoto Y, Oshima Y, Miki A, Wakabayashi T, Song D, Matsushita K, Hamasaki T,
      Nishida K. Clinical outcomes and changes in aqueous vascular endothelial growth
      factor levels after intravitreal bevacizumab for iris neovascularization and neovascu-
      lar glaucoma: a retrospective two-dose comparative study. J Ocul Pharmacol Ther
      2012;28:41-8.

[61] Shiba T, Sato Y, Takahashi M. Relationship between diabetic retinopathy and sleep-
      disordered breathing. Am J Ophthalmol. 2009 Jun;147(6):1017-21.

[62] Shiba T, Takahashi M, Hori Y, Saishin Y, Sato Y, Maeno T. Relationship between
      sleep-disordered breathing and iris and/or angle neovascularization in proliferative
      diabetic retinopathy cases. Am J Ophthalmol. 2011 Apr;151(4):604-9.

[63] Sinclair SH, Aaberg TM, Meredith TA. A pars plana filtering procedure combined
      with lensectomy and vitrectomy for neovascular glaucoma. Am J Ophthalmol
      1982;93:185-191.

[64] Singh Hayareh Sohan. Neovascular Glaucoma. Progress in Retinal and Eye Reaserch. 2007; 26: 470-480.

[65] Sohan Singh Hayreh. Neovascular Glaucoma. Prog Retin Eye Res. 2007 September ; 26(5): 470485.

[66] Stephen H. Sinclair, Evangelos S. Gragoudas. Prognosis for rubeosis iridis following central retinal vein occlusion. British Journal of Ophthalmology, 1979, 63, 735-743

[67] Teich SA, Walsh JB. A grading system for iris neovascularization. Prognostic implications for treatment. Ophthalmology,1981. 1102-6.

[68] The Diabetic Retinopathy Study Research Group. Preliminary report on effects of photocoagulation therapy. Am J Ophthalmol 1976;81:383-396.

[69] Torres-Soriano M, Reyna-Castelan E, Hernandez Rojas M, et al. Tractional retinal detachment after intravitreal injection of bevacizumab in proliferative diabetic retinopathy. Retin Cases Brief Rep 2009;3:70-73.

[70] Tripathi. Ramesh, MD. PhD. L. Junping, MD. PhD. Tripathi. Brenda, PhD. Chalekam. KV, MD. Adamis. Anthony P MD. Increased Levels of Vascular Endothelial Growth Factor in Aqueous Humor of Patients with Neovascular Glaucoma. Ophthalmology 1998; 105: 232-237

[71] Velez-Montoya R, Guerrero-Naranjo JL, Gonzalez-Mijares CC, Fromow-Guerra J, Marcellino GR, Quiroz-Mercado H, Morales-Cantón V.Pattern scan laser photocoagulation: safety and complications, experience after 1301 consecutive cases. Br J Ophthalmol 2010;94:720-4.

[72] Villarroel, M., Ciudin, A., Hernández, C. and Simo, R. (2010). Neurodegeneration: An early event of diabetic retinopathy. World J. Diabetes 15, 57-64.

[73] Wakabayashi T, Oshima Y, Sakaguchi H, Ikuno Y, Miki A, Gomi F, Otori Y, Kamei M, Kusaka S, Tano Y. Intravitreal bevacizumab to treat iris neovascularization and neovascular glaucoma secondary to ischemic retinal diseases in 41 consecutive cases. Ophthalmology 2008;115:1571-80.

[74] Wang Xiaoqin, Wang Guibo, Wang Yi. Intravitreous Vascular Endothelial Growth Factor and Hypoxia-Inductible Factor 1a in Patients with Proliferaive Diabetic Retinopathy. Am J Ophthalmol 2009; 148: 883-889.

[75] Will Whitmire, Mohammed MH Al-Gayyary, Mohammed Abdelsaid,Bilal K Yousufzai, Azza B El-Remessy. Alteration of growth factors and neuronal death in diabetic retinopathy: what we have learned so far. Molecular Vision 2011; 17:300-308

[76] Wittström E, Holmberg H, Hvarfner C, Andréasson S. Clinical and electrophysiologic outcome in patients with neovascular glaucoma treated with and without bevacizumab. Eur J Ophthalmol 2012;22:563-74.

[77] Yazdani S, Hendi K, Pakravan M, Mahdavi M, Yaseri M. Intravitreal bevacizumab for neovascular glaucoma: a randomized controlled trial. J Glaucoma 2009;18:632-7.

[78] Yoshida N, Hisatomi T, Ikeda Y, Kohno R, Murakami Y, Imaki H, Ueno A, Fujisawa K, Ishibashi T. Intravitreal bevacizumab treatment for neovascular glaucoma: histopathological analysis of trabeculectomy specimens. Graefes Arch Clin Exp Ophthalmol 2011;249:1547-52.

Chapter 3

Cornea and Glaucoma

Gema Bolivar, Javier Paz Moreno-Arrones and
Miguel A. Teus

Additional information is available at the end of the chapter

1. Introduction

Glaucoma is an acquired optic neuropathy in which destruction of ganglion cells and fibers leads to irreversible visual field loss. The prevalence of glaucoma, a leading cause of visual impairment and blindness worldwide [1,2], in the general population is about 2%. Increased intraocular pressure (IOP) is a primary risk factor for glaucoma development. IOP evaluation is used to assess disease control and treatment response, and lowering IOP has resulted in reducing the rates of disease progression over 5 years [3-7]. These data confirmed that elevated IOP is a pathophysiologic basis for glaucoma; therefore, accurate IOP measurement is critical in glaucoma.

Goldmann applanation tonometry (GAT), the gold standard for measuring IOP, estimates the IOP based on the force needed to flatten the corneal apex to a diameter of 3.06 mm. This area was chosen empirically to offset the surface tension of the tear film, which tends to draw the tonometry tip toward the eye, and the corneal and ocular rigidity, which affect the applanation force needed independent of the IOP level. When applanating this area, a gravitational force of 0.1 g corresponds to an IOP of 1 mmHg. Goldmann and Schmidt [8] found that when large variations in the central corneal thickness (CCT) occur, the accuracy of the GAT values can be affected.

The corneal rigidity affects the IOP measurements. The corneal biomechanics are more complex than central pachymetry alone and include viscosity, bioelasticity, hydration, regional pachymetry, and likely other as yet undetermined factors [9,10].

2. Corneal anatomy and histology

The cornea, the primary refractive ocular structure that contributes to focusing the external images on the retina, measures 11 to 12 mm horizontally, 10 to 11 mm vertically, and is about 0.5 mm thick centrally. The corneal thickness increases gradually toward the periphery to about 0.7 mm. Corneal nutrition depends on both glucose diffusing from the aqueous humor and oxygen supplied from the air through the tear film and in the peripheral cornea from the limbal blood vessels [11]. The cornea accounts for more than two thirds of the total ocular refractive power. Any slight change in the corneal contour can cause a substantial change in the ocular refractive power. The corneal optical properties are determined by its transparency, surface smoothness, contour, and refractive index.

The cornea is comprised of five layers: the epithelium, Bowman's layer, stroma, Descemet's membrane, and endothelium. The epithelium, the most anterior layer, is comprised of non-keratinizing stratified squamous epithelial cells. The epithelium and tear film form an optically smooth surface. The Bowman's layer is the most anterior part of the corneal stroma, and is adjacent to the epithelial basement membrane.

The structural and optical features depend mainly on the structure and composition of the corneal stroma, which represents up to 90% of the corneal thickness. Corneal transparency basically depends on the regular spacial distribution of the stromal cells and the stromal lamellae, and also on the water content of the stroma, that must be kept at a constant level of about 78%. The keratocytes are highly scattered and do not affect transparency. The lattice structure of the corneal collagen fibers, within a distance of 0.5 microns of the visible wavelength, is responsible for corneal transparency. Any decrease (dehydration) or increase (edema) in this distance results in a loss of transparency. Fibrillar collagen types I and V, which are intertwined with type VI collagen filaments (collagen types III, XII, and XIV have also been found in the stroma) and corneal proteoglycans (mainly decorin associated with dermatan sulfate and lumican associated with keratan sulfate), are the fundamental components of the extracellular matrix (ECM).

Negatively charged stromal glycosaminoglycans tend to repel each other, producing the corneal swelling pressure (SP) (of about 50 mmHg in the excised cornea), and can absorb and retain large amounts of water. The keratocytes lie between the corneal lamellae and synthesize both collagen and proteoglycans.

The diameter of each collagen fiber and the distance between the collagen fibers are homogeneous and measure less than half of the wavelength of the visible light (400-700 nm). This anatomic distribution of fibers is responsible for the fact that the incident light rays scattered by each collagen fiber are cancelled by the interference of other scattered rays, which allows the incident light to pass through the cornea without optical disruption.

Descemet's membrane, the basement membrane of the endothelium, is highly elastic and can withstand high pressure. When injured, it can regenerate.

The endothelium, the innermost corneal layer, is a monolayer of hexagonally shaped endothelial cells arranged in a mosaic pattern. The integrity of this layer and the correct function of the endothelial pump, which is linked to the ion-transport system controlled by enzymes such as Na^+, K^+-ATPase, are necessary to maintain the stability of the corneal water content. Therefore, the endothelium prevents corneal edema by both the barrier and the pump functions. The pump function generates the so-called corneal imbibition pressure (IP), a negative pressure that draws fluid into the cornea. The IP is equal to the SP in the excised cornea. In vivo, however, the IP is lower than the SP because of the compressive effect of the IOP on the cornea. The relationship between these three parameters is described by the equation:

$$IP = IOP - SP \tag{1}$$

Although the regulation of the corneal hydration is maintained largely by the function of the endothelial pump, the epithelial barrier effect, the surface evaporation, the IOP level, and the SP also play a role.

3. Impact of CCT on tonometry

The Ocular Hypertension Treatment Study (OHTS) [13] was a multicenter, randomized, prospective clinical trial of the efficacy of topical ocular hypotensive medications in delaying or preventing glaucoma onset in patients with ocular hypertension (OHT). Based on the OHTS, the CCT measured by pachymetry (Figure 1) has become important in glaucoma, and the study showed that the CCT is a significant predictor of the patients with OHT who are at higher risk of developing glaucoma, with a hazard ratio of 1.82 for each 40-μm thinning of the CCT.

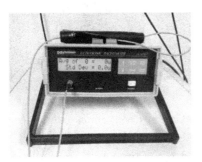

Figure 1. Ultrasound Pachymeter DGH 500 (Pachette™)

Eyes with a CCT of 555 μm or less had a three-fold greater risk of developing glaucoma compared with eyes that had a CCT exceeding 588 μm. In the multivariate model of baseline characteristics predictive of conversion oh OHT to glaucoma, the CCT had the greatest impact on the risk. These findings were confirmed in the European Glaucoma Prevention Study [14].

The CCT can be easily and accurately measured, it remains quite constant over a patient's lifetime, and, thus, just one CCT measurement is adequate in most patients. It is not clear why the CCT is such a strong predictor of the development of primary open-angle glaucoma (POAG) in OHT patients. In a multivariable model including age, baseline GAT IOP, optic disc topography (cup to disc [c/d] ratio), and visual field (pattern standard deviation [PSD]), although the CCT and IOP have independent effects on the risk of developing POAG, the two factors interact. Nevertheless, because GAT measurements depend on the CCT, it was impossible in the original model to completely disassociate the effects of both. These findings prove that CCT is an independent risk factor for glaucoma development. The CCT artifacts the GAT, so the IOP may be overestimated or underestimated in thick or thin corneas, respectively.

In 1975, Ehlers cannulated 29 eyes undergoing cataract surgery and found differences between the cannulated IOP and GAT IOP that were related to the CCT [15]; the GAT IOP was most accurate when the CCT was 520 μm. These results indicated that the CCT varies among individuals, and that this variations significantly affect the GAT IOP (Figure 2); therefore, deviations from the 520-μm reference value produced under- and overestimates of 7 mmHg for every 100 μm of deviation.

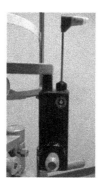

Figure 2. Goldmann applanation tonometer on a slit-lamp.

Investigators have attempted to design nomograms or correction formulas to account for the effect of CCT on GAT-IOP measurement [15-18], but none has been satisfactory.

The use of the available formulas to obtain a CCT-corrected GAT IOP does not improve the accuracy of the models to predict the risk of glaucoma development [19]. The predictive abilities were similar between the original OHTS model that included CCT, and other models that did not include the CCT but only the CCT-corrected IOP. This may mean that the CCT is relatively unimportant in the final predictive ability of the multivariable model as long as the CCT-corrected IOP is included. For example, a model including the IOP values corrected by the Ehlers formula [15] (a commonly used CCT correction formula that excluded the CCT) had a predictive ability almost identical to the original OHTS model. Such a result could hardly indicate a major true independent contribution of CCT as a prognostic factor of glaucoma development.

The fundamental concept supporting this correction formula is that as corneas become thinner, the GAT measurements become too low. If the CCT is an average value, the GAT value is essentially correct, and if the cornea is thicker than average, the GAT overvalues the true manometric IOP. Although the Ehlers formula was based on manometric data, the weakness of the formula arises from the small number of subjects studied and the high degree of variability among the subjects. Ehler's data showed a tendency for the Goldmann IOP to increase with increasing CCTs; however, a close look at that data indicates that many subjects clearly defy that trend, i.e., the Goldmann values were too low in some subjects with thick corneas and too high in some with thin corneas. The correlations between the IOP and CCT with Ehler's data and data from similar studies are too low to allow definitive clinical decision-making based on these formulas. However, adjusting the IOP using CCT-based formulas has resulted in poorer agreement with Pascal dynamic contour tonometry, a slit-lamp mounted tonometer for measuring IOP wich seems to be independent of the corneal properties (Figure 3), compared with unadjusted GAT IOP values [20]. It suggested that, although the CCT may be useful in population analyses, CCT-based correction formulas should not be applied to individuals.

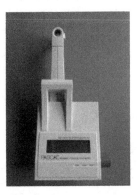

Figure 3. Dinamic contour tonometer.

CCT correction formulas for GAT measurements are probably of little value in clinical practice [21]. It might be advantageous to incorporate the risk information from validated predictive models of glaucoma development or progression [19,21], so clinicians have to account for baseline older age, higher IOP, larger vertical c/d ratio, thinner CCT, and greater PSD in the visual field. The hypothesis that CCT is a true independent risk factor for glaucoma is currently not validated and requires further investigation.

In addition, the CCT is becoming more important clinically because of the large number of patients who undergo laser in situ keratomileusis (LASIK), which causes high IOP elevations intraoperatively [22] and a permanent corneal thinning, that, therefore, affects the IOP evaluation.

Because the IOP is an important risk factor for glaucoma, accurate measurement is important, and it can be achieved by intraocular manometry; however, this is an invasive method that obviously cannot be used in a clinical setting,

The only way to fully evaluate the possible independent role of CCT as a prognostic factor for glaucoma development is to include in the predictive model the IOP measurements obtained by a CCT-independent tonometer. The Pascal dynamic contour tonometer (DCT), is a slit-lamp-mounted, nonapplanation, digital contact tonometer that provides continuous tonometry recordings that measure the IOP and the ocular pulse amplitude, which is the difference between the minimal and maximal values of the pulsatile IOP wave contour, and does not require corneal applanation and the DCT IOP measurements seem to agree closely with manometric measurements [23]. Therefore, including DCT measurements with the CCT in a predictive model for glaucoma might better assess the true independent value of CCT compared with use of only the CCT-corrected GAT values. This has been investigated in patients undergoing phacoemulsification, that had the anterior chamber cannulated in a closed system and the IOP was set to 15, 20, and 35 mmHg by a water column. The IOP measurements then were taken by DCT. The results showed that the DCT agree well with the intracameral IOP. Interestingly, the CCT had a low but significant effect on the DCT measurements [23].

The DCT measurement principle is based on contour matching, which assumes that if the eye were enclosed by a contoured, tight-fitting shell, the forces generated by IOP would act on the shell wall. Replacing part of the shell wall with a pressure sensor would enable measurement of these forces and therefore the IOP. The DCT has a central gauge surrounded by a contoured plastic tip that is in contact with the cornea and creates a tight-fitting shell. The DCT compensates for all forces exerted on the cornea and an electronic sensor measures IOP independent of the corneal properties.

4. Corneal thickness and glaucoma

Most of the knowledge regarding the impact of corneal thickness in glaucoma is referred to CCT; however, Jordan et al. [24] found differences between the OHT and normal tension glaucoma (NTG) groups in central and paracentral corneal thicknesses measured by optical slip scan pachymetry. The study corroborated differences in CCT between OHT and NTG but also found that the corresponding paracentral quadrants differed significantly between groups. Patients with NTG had overall thinner corneas and those with OHT had overall thicker corneas. Is the corneal thickness an independent risk factor for glaucoma?

Goldmann first suggested in 1957 that the IOP measured by applanation tonometry might be affected by the CCT [25]. He found that IOP measurements in patients with thin corneas tended to be underestimated but overestimated in those with thick corneas.

In the OHTS, the GAT IOP was used to determine participant eligibility, guide treatment decisions, and construct a model predictive of POAG development. Had the OHTS been carried out with a perfectly accurate, cornea-independent tonometer, which does not exist, the IOP might have been a more powerful predictor of POAG development and the CCT might have been a less powerful predictor. Some investigators interpreted the OHTS results to indicate that the CCT is an independent risk factor for glaucoma development. Because the GAT measurements ultimately depend on the CCT, Medeiros and Weinreb [26] stated that it is impossible, based on the original model, to disassociate the effects of both. Some groups have evaluated [19,27,28] whether the OHTS prediction model could be improved using CCT-corrected IOP using previously published formulas (Table 1), evaluated using the c statistics (a measure of concordance), and calibration chi-squares. The c statistic is the fraction of patients with an outcome among pairs of patients, in which one has the outcome and one does not; the patient with the higher predictive value is classified as the one with the outcome. The c statistic varies between 0.5 when a model provides no information and 1.0 in sensible models. The CCT also remained a significant predictor of glaucoma development in a multivariable model that included the CCT-corrected IOP.

CCT in microns	IOP correction in mm Hg
445	7
455	6
465	6
475	5
485	4
495	4
505	3
515	2
525	1
535	1
545	0
555	-1
565	-1
575	-2
585	-3
595	-4
605	-4
615	-5
625	-6
635	-6
645	-7

Table 1. Correction values for IOPs based on CCT [8,17].

Medeiros and Weinreb [26] argued that other factors besides corneal thickness such as corneal elasticity and viscoelasticity might affect tonometric readings and the formulas to correct the GAT IOP [19] do not fully consider these factors [19, 27, 28]. The DCT measurements have been proposed and agree closely with the manometric measurements [20]. Therefore, the inclusion of DCT measurements along with corneal thickness in a model predictive of glaucoma might better assess the true independent value of IOP. A biologic link might exist between some corneal parameters such as the thickness or the viscoelastic properties and the structure/deformability/physiology of the lamina cribosa and peripapillary sclera.

It is noteworthy that in the Early Manifest Glaucoma Trial (EMGT) the IOP was not used to determine patient eligibility or treatment decisions, and thus the possible effect of the CCT on GAT measurements was less likely to affect the incidence of glaucoma progression. In the EMGT, the CCT was an independent factor predictive of POAG progression [29]. In the population-based, longitudinal Barbados Eye Studies, the CCT (measured 9 years after the recruitment) was an independent risk factor for development of glaucoma [30]. In the population-based Los Angeles Latino Eye Study (LALES), the prevalence of glaucoma was higher among individuals with thin CCTs than among individuals with normal or thick CCTs across all IOP levels [31]. The LALES, which investigated whether adjusting each IOP individually for CCT using the Doughty and Zaman algorithm [16] changed this relationship, reported almost no change in the association between a thin CCT and a higher prevalence of glaucoma. This algorithm showed that 2.5 mmHg was correlated with a 50-µm difference from the baseline CCT. Each of these corrective factors had proponents, and the use of algorithms to correct for the IOP based on the CCT became popular. The LALES concluded that the CCT is an independent factor itself [31]. The findings of the EMGT, Barbados Eye Studies, and LALES suggest that the effect of CCT on the glaucoma development risk is caused by more than just a tonometry artifact.

5. Corneal biomechanics

Ocular biomechanics is an increasingly important field. Overt corneal biomechanical problems have long been seen in keratoconus and corneal ectasia after corneal refractive surgery [32].

In keratoconus, there are clear changes in the corneal collagen, and the cornea loses rigidity over time and becomes ectatic; in corneal ectasia, the ablation of some corneal stroma can weaken the cornea and result in progressive corneal deformation [33]. In refractive surgical practice, patients with preexisting ectasia usually are excluded from treatment. However, individual variations in biomechanical integrity and postoperative wound healing preclude preoperative identification of all potentially vulnerable patients. There is considerable but mostly indirect evidence suggesting that the biomechanical corneal properties vary with age. Quantifying the biomechanical corneal properties is difficult, but the available evidence supports corneal stiffening with age; in other words, there is an increment in Young's modulus [34], the ocular rigidity coefficient, that expresses the elastic properties of the globe [35,36], the cohesive tensile strength, and the breaking force of a tissue [37].

Young's modulus, also known as the tensile modulus, is a measure of the stiffness of an elastic material and is a parameter used to characterize elastic materials. Perhaps the single best descriptor of a given material's biomechanical properties at low strain is its Young's modulus (E), which is defined as the ratio of stress to strain or

$$Young's\ modulus(E) = stress\ /\ strain$$

where stress is an applied force (load/unit area), and strain is the deformation of the material to which stress has been applied (displacement/unit length). This parameter depends on the material's physical properties and dimensions. Importantly, when stress is applied and removed, elastic materials follow the same path during deformation and relaxation and ultimately recover the original shape. Viscoelastic materials, such as the cornea, also can recover the original shape after stress is removed, but the relaxation path differs from the deformation path; therefore, the relationship between stress and strain is nonlinear, and stiffening occurs as strain increases [38-40] (Figure 4). This behavior, referred to as corneal hysteresis (CH), results from dissipation of energy as heat in the material.

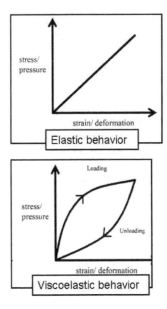

Figure 4. Here, it can be seen the relationship between stress and strain is linear in an elastic behaviour and nonlinear in a viscoelastic behaviour.

The GAT IOP measurement, obtained from the force needed to applanate the cornea, is based on a number of assumptions about corneal deformability. The corneal mix of collagen types, corneal hydration, collagen fibril density, ECM, and other factors vary among individuals. In some patients, these factors dwarf the effect of the CCT on the accuracy of the GAT IOP value. In fact, the effect of the corneal thickness on GAT measurements may be less important than the effect of variations in corneal elasticity [41].

CH is a measure of the viscoelastic properties of the corneal tissue together with the corneal resistance factor (CRF), i.e., the "energy absorption capability" of the cornea, and indicates the biomechanical integrity. The Ocular Response Analyzer (ORA) (Reichert Ophthalmic Instruments, Inc., Buffalo, NY) provides both parameters (Figure 5).

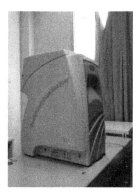

Figure 5. Ocular response analyzer.

The ORA, which measures some of the corneal biomechanical properties in vivo, uses a 25-millisencond (ms) air pulse to apply pressure to the cornea. The air pulse causes the cornea to move inward, past applanation and into a slight concavity, before returning to the normal curvature. Corneal deformation is recorded via an electro-optical infrared detection system similar to classic air-puff tonometry. The ORA acquires corneal biomechanical data by quantifying this differential inward and outward corneal response to the air pulse over about 20 ms (Figure 6).

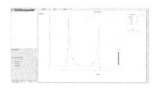

Figure 6. This picture shows the measurements done by ORA.

Because of the dynamic nature of the measurement process, viscous damping in the cornea causes delays in the inward and outward applanation events (energy absorption). Milliseconds after the first applanation, the air pump that generated the air pulse also shuts down, and the air pressure applied to the eye decreases in an inverse-time symmetric fashion. However, before that decrease, the cornea is indented substantially as the air pressure peaks about 3 ms after applanation. As the pressure decreases from its peak, the cornea passes through a second applanated state while returning to the normal convex curvature. This allows detection of a second applanation point. Using the first applanation pressure point (P1) and the second applanation pressure point (P2) [42,43] (Figure 7), the ORA generates two separate IOP output parameters, and the difference between the two pressures is CH.

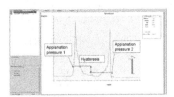

Figure 7. This picture shows de P1 and P2 points. Hysteresis is also showed.

The Goldmann-correlated IOP (IOPg) is the average of the inward (P1) and outward (P2) applanation pressures. This parameter is closely correlated with the GAT IOP.

The CH measurement also provides a basis for two additional new parameters: the corneal-compensated IOP (IOPcc), an IOP measurement that is less affected by corneal properties than other tonometric methods, such as GAT, and CRF, an index of corneal resistance to deformation derived from the formula P1 x kP2, where k is the constant determined from empirical analysis of the relationship between both P1 and P2 and CCT to develop a corneal parameter more strongly associated with CCT than CH [44].

The CH in patients with glaucoma and in those with acquired optic nerve head (ONH) pits is lower than in normal controls [43, 45]. Other authors also have found that the CH predicts visual field damage progression. However, other studies using the ORA have reported that the CRF and CH did not change significantly when the IOP was lowered using topical anti-glaucoma drugs and that the relationship between the GAT IOP and CRF or CH is weak and unchanged by ocular hypotensive drugs [46].

6. Corneal and refractive surgeries

The changes in the GAT IOP after corneal refractive surgery have been studied because of the large number of patients who undergo laser refractive procedures. In corneal laser excimer refractive surgery, the cornea becomes thinner and, therefore, the IOP measurement is affected [47,48]. Because most patients undergoing laser refractive surgery are myopic and at increased risk for glaucoma [28], the effect of these procedures on glaucoma management should be determined.

After laser ablation, the corneal thickness and shape change, so the mathematical assumptions used in existing models for IOP measurement cannot be satisfied [49]. In lamellar procedures, creation of a corneal flap changes the corneal biomechanical stability. The depth-dependent tensile strength of the cornea, also have been reported [50,51], with the anterior 40% of stroma having a significantly higher tensile strength than the posterior 60%; therefore, a corneal flap can have viscoelastic properties that differ from the underlying stroma and further affect the GAT IOP readings. Patients who underwent LASIK and laser-assisted subepithelial keratomileusis seem to have a postoperative decrease in CH [52,53].

In some cases, LASIK is associated with the interface fluid syndrome (IFS), first described by Rehany et al. [54], that is characterized by fluid collection in the flap interface due to a marked IOP increase. The resultant GAT IOP value is falsely lower [48]. In normal corneas with intact functioning membranes and avascular compact corneal stroma, the stroma bears the acute IOP increases, and the fluid flows from the stroma to the epithelium, which has lower pressure, resulting in epithelial edema. After LASIK, there is a virtual space between the flap and the stromal bed, with fluid accumulating in the flap interface [55].

7. Cornea, lamina cribrosa, and glaucoma

The lamina cribrosa is a sieve-like fenestrated structure in the posterior sclera through which the optic nerve fibers and the retinal vessels enter and exit the eye. The glial segment of the optic nerve and lamina cribrosa derive from the neuroectoderm, and the mesenchyme originates from the neural crest. Because the corneal stroma and the corneal endothelium also derive from the neural crest, they are related embryologically. The lamina cribrosa is believed to be the site at which the neural damage induced by glaucoma occurs.

The CCT may reflect the scleral and lamina cribrosa properties associated with glaucomatous optic neuropathy. In fact, the CCT is correlated with the anterior scleral thickness in patients with POAG [56]. Several studies have assessed the relationship between the CCT and objectively measured optic disc parameters, but they provide inconsistent results. Using the confocal scanning laser ophthalmoscopy (Heidelberg Retina Tomograph, Heidelberg Engineering, Heidelberg, Germany), several hospital-based studies of patients with glaucoma have suggested that the CCT is correlated with the optic disc area and nasal rim volume [57], while another population-based study [58] did not identify these correlations. In another population-based survey [59], no significant relationship was found between the CCT and ONH parameters obtained with retinal tomography.

Thin corneas also can be associated with weak ONHs and this weakness may be related with a thin lamina cribrosa [60-62]. Further, the development and progression of glaucoma are correlated with the CCT [62]. Other studies have suggested that CH and not corneal thickness is correlated with the vulnerability of the ONH to sustain glaucomatous damage [63].

The correlation between CCT and ONH topographic changes in response to IOP reductions in patients with POAG also has been evaluated [64]. The hypothesis was that thinner CCTs might be associated with greater changes in ONH topography due to a more compliant lamina cribrosa. Nicolela et al. [65] found that patients with thinner corneas show significantly greater cup shallowing, which is a surrogate marker for lamina cribrosa displacement and compliance in response to IOP reduction. The investigators interrupted the medical treatment for 4 weeks (with an average increase of IOP of 5.4 mmHg), and when the medical treatment was restarted, the IOPs were remeasured after 4 weeks, and they found that the IOP decreased from a mean of 22.27±4.12 mmHg to a mean of 17.39±2.67 mmHg. This finding may support the hypothesis that eyes with a thinner CCT have an increased risk of developing glaucomatous ONH changes because the lamina cribrosa may be more prone to displacement in response to IOP changes. Nevertheless, the changes of the ONH topography were unconfirmed [65] for relatively moderate IOP changes of about 5 mmHg. In addition, the stage of the ONH glaucomatous damage and the disease duration might affect the degree of compliance of the lamina in response to IOP changes, so that for more advanced and long-standing damage less compliance of the lamina can be expected.

The differences in laminar thickness have been studied in different glaucoma types. Park et al. [66] reported that NTG was associated with a thinner lamina cribrosa than OAG in patients with a similar disease stage; another study showed that patients with pseudoexfoliation syndrome have less stiffness compared with normal controls, which may reflect an inherent tissue weakness that makes these eyes more vulnerable to glaucomatous damage [67].

Researchers generally agree that the lamina cribrosa is important in glaucoma [68]. Nevertheless, in vivo clinical clues regarding the correlated parameters of the lamina cribrosa are limited [69, 70].

8. Effect of topical hypotensive drugs on the cornea

Some ocular hypotensive drugs, such as topical carbonic anhydrase inhibitors (CAIs) and F2α-prostaglandin analogs (PGAs), induce changes in the CCT [71].

The hypotensive effect of PGAs, first-line treatments of glaucoma and OHT, may be affected by some ocular characteristics, such as the axial length [72]. Eyes with a longer axial length have a worse response to PGAs treatment. If a patient had undergone a previous argon laser trabeculoplasty, there is a minimal response to a PGA [73]. In addition to its effectiveness in lowering IOP, PGAs have mild and local side effects that include changes in iris color in up to 70% of patients [74], especially in patients with mixed colors and in the irises of older patients [75]. The changes in iris pigmentation are related to increased melanin content of the iris melanocytes [76]. Other side effects are periocular hyperpigmentation and darkening and increased eyelash length. PGAs are highly efficient for lowering IOP, with few local and systemic side effects. Interestingly, most recent studies have shown that PGAs decrease the CCT, and Viestenz et al. [77] reported thinner CCTs in patients treated with topical prostaglandin F2-alpha, compared with topical CAIs. Harasymowycz et al. in a prospective study

[78] found a mean 6.9-micron CCT decrease after 6 weeks of travoprost treatment. Sen et al. [79] reported $1.9 \pm 2.4\%$ and $2.8 \pm 1.8\%$ CCT decreases over 24 months with latanoprost and bimatoprost, respectively. Hatanaka et al. [80] also reported that topical PGAs were associated with a CCT reduction over at least 8 weeks (the bimatoprost 0.03% group decreased from 544.41 ± 35.4 to 540.35 ± 35.9 μm; the travoprost 0.004% group decreased from 538.47 ± 32.0 to 532.25 ± 30.4 μm; the latanoprost 0.005% group decreased from 548.57 ± 32.4 to 543.88 ± 35.6 μm). Zhong et al. [81] reported CCT reductions in the latanoprost, travoprost, and bimatoprost groups of 14.95 ± 5.04, 15.73 ± 3.25, and 17.00 ± 6.23 mm, respectively, and no significant difference was seen in the CCT reductions between patients with 6 months or shorter treatment and patients with 6 months or longer treatment in the three groups.

The reason for the effect of the PGAs on the CCT is unknown, but it is widely accepted that PGAs seem to induce ECM remodeling due to a FP-receptor-mediated increased synthesis of matrix metalloproteinases (MMPs) [82]. The MMPs are a family of enzymes that degrade several components of the ECM, thus decreasing the levels of collagen types I, II, III, and IV. Published evidence suggests that the PGA-related activation of the MMPs activity takes place in the ciliary body, the trabecular meshwork [83], the conjunctiva, the sclera, and the zonular fibers-ciliary muscle complex [84]. Further, naturally occurring prostaglandins seem to play a relevant role in physiologic corneal conditions, i.e., repair after corneal injuries, and in pathologic corneal conditions, i.e., corneal ectasia. In fact, PGA treatment may be related to keratoconus progression [85]. Thus, there is enough evidence to suggest that topical PGAs might induce changes in the ECM of the corneal stroma via up-regulation of MMPs that may slightly change the CCT and perhaps the corneal viscoelastic properties. In fact, CH seems to be significantly lower in PGA-treated eyes [86]. PGAs also seem to increase the keratocyte density in the corneal stroma, which might also result in changes in the ECM [87].

Previous reports have suggested that chronic topical PGA treatment is associated with a slight decrease in the CCT [86,88] and an increase in the CH. We studied the response of CCT to increased IOP in rabbit eyes treated with travoprost for 1 month and in an untreated control group, and found that the decrease in CCT induced by a sudden increase in IOP was greater in the PGA-treated eyes than in the control eyes [88]. The changes in corneal thickness induced by IOP increases are believed to be a strain response and thus are probably a biomechanical response of the corneal tissue to the IOP changes. Then the differences in the CCT behavior between groups also suggest that PGAs induce changes in the corneal biomechanical properties, at least in rabbits.

Topical dorzolamide induces a 14.4% increase in CCT in patients with corneal guttata [89]. Patients with severe corneal guttata or a highly compromised endothelial function may have a higher risk of corneal decompensation after prolonged topical use of dorzolamide.

Dorzolamide is a potent cytosolic carbonic anhydrase inhibitor (CAI) isoenzyme II, and the corneal endothelium contains carbonic anhydrase (CA) II and the cytosolic CA I, which plays a major role in keeping the cornea relatively dehydrated. Dorzolamide has a high affinity for CA II and low affinity for CA I, and thus, it has the potential to interfere with the pump function of the corneal endothelium, which could theoretically lead to corneal edema. Changes in CCT have been used as an indirect indicator of the endothelial function. Some investigations have reported a slight but significant increase in CCT in eyes treated with brinzolamide, another CAI inhibitor [90]. Another way to measure the endothelial function in vivo is to measure the intrastromal corneal pressure [91,92], formerly known as corneal intrastromal pressure, which has a negative value under physiologic conditions. The amount of negative pressure in the corneal stroma is likely to be correlated with the endothelial function, and topical dorzolamide significantly reduces the negative pressure in the corneal stroma in rabbits [91], suggesting that the drug affects the endothelial function in healthy rabbit corneas. This finding is consistent with the reported cases of dorzolamide-induced corneal edema in susceptible patients and with the finding that inhibiting CA in the corneal endothelium causes a 50% decrease in the endothelial fluid transport and some corneal swelling [92].

9. Conclusion

There is growing interest in the possible effect of some corneal parameters in glaucoma. There is sufficient evidence to suggest that CCT evaluation predicts the risk of conversion from OHT to glaucoma. The influence of the CCT on the GAT IOP is clear, so true IOP is higher than GAT IOP in patients with thinner corneas and true IOP is lower than GAT IOP in patients with thicker corneas. In addition, some data suggest that CCT may be an independent risk factor for glaucoma development, although there is no clear evidence to support this hypothesis.

Of special interest is the fact that GAT is affected by laser excimer refractive surgery, a popular procedure that changes some corneal properties that affect accurate IOP measurement. New tonometers with a lower relationship to the corneal thickness and viscoelastic properties need to be developed.

Finally, widely used topical antiglaucomatous medications can alter the corneal viscoelastic properties and thus affect the GAT readings. This also needs to be investigated further.

Author details

Gema Bolivar[1], Javier Paz Moreno-Arrones[1*] and Miguel A. Teus[2]

*Address all correspondence to: javierpazmoreno@gmail.com

1 Department of Glaucoma, Hospital Universitario Príncipe de Asturias, Alcalá de Henares, Spain

2 Department of Ophthalmology, Hospital Universitario Príncipe de Asturias, University of Alcalá, Alcalá de Henares, Spain

References

[1] Congdon N, O'Colmain B, Klaver CC, et al. Causes and prevalence of visual impairment among adults in the United States. Arch Ophthalmol 2004;122(4):477– 485.

[2] Friedman DS, Wolfs RC, O'Colmain BJ, et al. Prevalence of open-angle glaucoma among adults in the United States. Arch Ophthalmol 2004;122(4):532–538.

[3] Kass MA, Heuer DK, Higginbotham EJ, et al. The Ocular Hypertension Treatment Study: a randomized trial determines that topical ocular hypotensive medication delays or prevents the onset of primary open-angle glaucoma. Arch Ophthalmol 2002;120(6):701–713, discussion 829-830.

[4] Collaborative Initial Normal-Tension Glaucoma Study Group. Comparison of glaucomatous progression between untreated patients with normal-tension glaucoma and patients with therapeutically reduced intraocular pressures. Am J Ophthalmol 1998;126(4):487– 497.

[5] Aoyama A, Ishida K, Sawada A, Yamamoto T. Target intraocular pressure for stability of visual field loss progression in normal-tension glaucoma. Jpn J Ophthalmol. 2010 Mar;54(2):117-23. Epub 2010 Apr 18.

[6] The Advanced Glaucoma Intervention Study (AGIS): 7. The relationship between control of intraocular pressure and visual field deterioration. Am J Ophthalmol 2000; 130(4):429–440.

[7] Heijl A, Leske MC, Bengtsson B, et al. Reduction of intraocular pressure and glaucoma progression: results from the Early Manifest Glaucoma Trial. Arch Ophthalmol 2002; 120(10):1268 –1279.

[8] Doughty MJ, Zaman ML. Human corneal thickness and its impact on intraocular pressure measures: a review and metaanalysis approach. Surv Ophthalmol 2000;44(5):367– 408.

[9] Liu J, Roberts CJ. Influence of corneal biomechanical properties on intraocular pressure measurement: quantitative analysis. J Cataract Refract Surg 2005;31(1):146 –155.

[10] Medeiros FA, Weinreb RN. Evaluation of the influence of corneal biomechanical properties on intraocular pressure measurements using the ocular response analyzer. J Glaucoma 2006;15(5):364 –370.

[11] Turss R, Schebitz H.Significance of the aqueous humor and marginal loop vessels for the nutrition of the cornea. Ber Zusammenkunft Dtsch Ophthalmol Ges. 1972;71:87-91.

[12] Bonanno JA. Molecular mechanisms underlying the corneal endothelial pump. Exp Eye Res. 2012 Feb;95(1):2-7.

[13] Lester M, Mete M, Figus M, Frezzotti P. Incorporating corneal pachymetry into the management of glaucoma. J Cataract Refract Surg. 2009 Sep;35(9):1623-8.

[14] Ocular Hypertension Treatment Study Group and the European Glaucoma Prevention Study Group. The accuracy and clinical application of predictive models for primary open-angle glaucoma in ocular hypertensive individuals.Ophthalmology. 2008 Nov;115(11):2030-6.

[15] Ehlers N, Bramsen T, Sperling S. Applanation tonometry and central corneal thickness. Acta Ophthalmol (Copenh) 1975; 53:34–43.

[16] Dueker DK, Singh K, Lin SC, Fechtner RD, Minckler DS, Samples JR, Schuman JS. Corneal thickness measurement in the management of primary open-angle glaucoma: a report by the American Academy of Ophthalmology. Ophthalmology. 2007 Sep;114(9):1779-87.

[17] Whitacre MM, Stein RA, Hassanein K. The effect of corneal thickness on applanation tonometry. Am J Ophthalmol 1993; 115:592– 6.

[18] Shimmyo M, Ross AJ, Moy A, Mostafavi R. Intraocular pressure, Goldmann applanation tension, corneal thickness, and corneal curvature in Caucasians, Asians, Hispanics, and African Americans. Am J Ophthalmol 2003;136:603–13.

[19] Brandt JD, Gordon MO, Gao F, et al. Adjusting intraocular pressure for central corneal thickness does not improve prediction models for primary open-angle glaucoma. Ophthalmology 2012;119:437– 42.

[20] Park SJ, Ang GS, Nicholas S, Wells AP. The effect of thin, thick, and normal corneas on Goldmann intraocular pressure measurements and correction formulae in individual eyes. Ophthalmology. 2012 Mar;119(3):443-9.

[21] Gordon MO, Torri V, Miglior S, et al. Validated prediction model for the development of primary open-angle glaucoma in individuals with ocular hypertension. Ophthalmology 2007; 114:10 –9.

[22] Hernandez-Verdejo JL, Teus MA, Roman JM, Bolivar G. Porcine model to compare real-time intraocular pressure during LASIK with a mechanical microkeratome and femtosecond laser. Invest Ophthalmol Vis Sci. 2007 Jan;48(1):68-72.

[23] Boehm AG, Weber A, Pillunat LE, et al. Dynamic contour tonometry in comparison to intracameral IOP measurements. Invest Ophthalmol Vis Sci 2008;49:2472–7.

[24] Jordan JF, Joergens S, Dinslage S, Dietlein TS, Krieglstein GK. Central and paracentral corneal pachymetry in patients with normal tension glaucoma and ocular hypertension. Graefes Arch Clin Exp Ophthalmol. 2006 Feb;244(2):177-82.

[25] Goldmann H, Schmidt T. Uber applanationstonometrie. Ophthalmologie 1957;134:221–42

[26] Medeiros FA, Weinreb RN. Is corneal thickness an independent risk factor for glaucoma? Ophthalmology. 2012 Mar;119(3):435-6.

[27] Brandt JD, Gordon MO, Beiser JA, Lin SC, Alexander MY, Kass MA. Changes in central corneal thickness over time: the ocular hypertension treatment study. Ocular Hypertension Treatment Study Group. Ophthalmology. 2008 Sep;115(9):1550-6, 1556

[28] Brandt JD. Central corneal thickness, tonometry, and glaucoma risk-a guide for the perplexed. Can J Ophthalmol. 2007 Aug;42(4):562-6.

[29] Leske MC, Heijl A, Hyman L, et al, EMGT Group. Predictors of long-term progression in the Early Manifest Glaucoma Trial. Ophthalmology 2007;114:1965–72.

[30] Leske MC, Wu SY, Hennis A, et al, BESs Study Group. Risk factors for incident open-angle glaucoma: the Barbados Eye Studies. Ophthalmology 2008;115:85–93.

[31] Francis BA, Varma R, Chopra V, et al, Los Angeles Latino Eye Study Group. Intraocular pressure, central corneal thickness, and prevalence of open-angle glaucoma: the Los Angeles Latino Eye Study. Am J Ophthalmol 2008;146:741– 6.

[32] Seiler T, Quurke AW. Iatrogenic keratectasia after LASIK in a case of forme fruste keratoconus. J Cataract Refract Surg. 1998;24: 1007–1009.

[33] Jaycock PD, Lobo L, Ibrahim J, Tyrer JR, Marshall J. Interferometric technique to measure biomechanical changes in the cornea induced by refractive surgery. J Cataract Refract Surg. 2005;31:175–184

[34] Elsheikh A, Wang D, Brown M, Rama P, Campanelli M, Pye D. Assessment of corneal biomechanical properties and their variation with age. Curr Eye Res. 2007;32:11–19.

[35] Ytteborg J. Further investigations of factors influencing size of rigidity coefficient. Acta Ophthalmologica. 1960;38:643–657.

[36] Pallikaris IG, Kymionis GD, Ginis HS, Kounis GA, Tsilimbaris MK. Ocular rigidity in living human eyes. Invest Ophthalmol Vis Sci. 2005;46:409–414.

[37] Randleman JB, Dawson DG, Grossniklaus HE, McCarey BE, Edelhauser HF. Depth-dependent cohesive tensile strength in human donor corneas: implications for refractive surgery. J Refract Surg. 2008;24:S85–89.

[38] Nyquist GW. Rheology of the cornea: experimental techniques and results. Exp Eye Res. 1968;7:183–188.

[39] Hjortdal JO. Extensibility of the normo-hydrated human cornea. Acta Ophthalmol Scand. 1995;73:12–17.

[40] Jue B, Maurice DM. The mechanical properties of the rabbit and human cornea. J Biomech. 1986;19:847–853

[41] Touboul D, Roberts C, Kérautret J, Garra C, Maurice-Tison S, Saubusse E, Colin J. Correlations between corneal hysteresis, intraocular pressure, and corneal central pachymetry. J Cataract Refract Surg. 2008 Apr;34(4):616-22.

[42] Kotecha A, White ET, Shewry JM, Garway-Heath DF. The relative effects of corneal thickness and age on Goldmann applanation tonometry and dynamic contour tonometry. Br J Ophthalmol. 2005 Dec;89(12):1572-5.

[43] Detry-Morel M, Jamart J, Pourjavan S. Evaluation of corneal biomechanical properties with the Reichert Ocular Response Analyzer. Eur J Ophthalmol. 2011 Mar-Apr; 21(2):138-48.

[44] Kotecha A. What biomechanical properties of the cornea are relevant for the clinician? Surv Ophthalmol. 2007 Nov;52 Suppl 2:S109-14.

[45] Bochmann F, Ang GS, Azuara-Blanco A. Lower corneal hysteresis in glaucoma patients with acquired pit of the optic nerve (APON). Graefes Arch Clin Exp Ophthalmol. 2008 Jan 12.

[46] Kotecha A, Elshkeikh A, Roberts CR, Zhu H, Garway-Heath DF. Properties of the cornea measured with the ocular response analyzer. Invest Ophthalmol Vis Sci 2006; 47: 5337-5347.

[47] Chatterjee A, Shah S, Bessant DA, Naroo SA, Doyle SJ. Reduction in intraocular pressure after excimer laser photorefractive keratectomy: correlation with pretreatment myopia. Ophthalmology 1997;104:355–359.

[48] Munger R, Hodge WG, Mintsioulis G, Agapitos PJ, Jackson WB, Damji KF. Correction of intraocular pressure for changes in central corneal thickness following photorefractive keratectomy. Can J Ophthalmol 1998;33:159 –165.

[49] Wells AP, Garway-Heath DF, Poostchi A, Wong T, Chan KC, Sachdev N. Corneal hysteresis but not corneal thickness correlates with optic nerve surface compliance in glaucoma patients. Invest Ophthalmol Vis Sci. 2008 Aug;49(8):3262-8.

[50] Randleman JB, Dawson DG, Grossniklaus HE, McCarey BE, Edelhauser HF. Depth-dependent cohesive tensile strength in human donor corneas: implications for refractive surgery. J Refract Surg 2008; 24:S85–S89

[51] Dawson DG, Grossniklaus HE, McCarey BE, Edelhauser HF. Biomechanical and wound healing characteristics of corneas after excimer laser keratorefractive surgery: is there a difference between advanced surface ablation and sub-Bowman's keratomileusis? J Refract Surg 2008; 24:S90–S96).

[52] Qazi MA, Sanderson JP, Mahmoud AM, Yoon EY, Roberts CJ, Pepose JS. Postoperative changes in intraocular pressure and corneal biomechanical metricsLaser in situ keratomileusis versus laser-assisted subepithelial keratectomy. J Cataract Refract Surg. 2009 Oct;35(10):1774-88.

[53] Kirwan C, O'Keefe M. Corneal hysteresis using the Reichert ocular response analyser: findings pre- andpost-LASIK and LASEK. Acta Ophthalmol. 2008 Mar;86(2): 215-8. Epub 2007 Sep 21.

[54] Rehany U, Bersudsky V, Rumelt S. Paradoxical hypotony after laser in situ keratomi-
      leusis. J Cataract Refract Surg. 2000 Dec;26(12):1823-6.

[55] Carreño E, Portero A, Galarreta DJ, Merayo JM.Interface fluid syndrome associated
      with cataract surgery. J Refract Surg. 2012 Apr;28(4):243-4.

[56] Mohamed-Noor J, Bochmann F, Siddiqui MA, Atta HR, Leslie T, Maharajan P, Wong
      YM, Azuara-Blanco A. Correlation between corneal and scleral thickness in glauco-
      ma. J Glaucoma. 2009 Jan;18(1):32-6.

[57] Terai N, Spoerl E, Pillunat LE, Kuhlisch E, Schmidt E, Boehm AG. The relationship
      between central corneal thickness and optic disc size in patients with primary open-
      angle glaucoma in a hospital-based population. Acta Ophthalmol. 2011 Sep;89(6):
      556-9.

[58] Tomidokoro A, Araie M, Iwase A; Tajimi Study Group. Corneal thickness and relat-
      ing factors in a population-based study in Japan: theTajimi study. Am J Ophthalmol.
      2007 Jul;144(1):152-4.

[59] Hawker MJ, Edmunds MR, Vernon SA, Hillman JG, MacNab HK. The relationship
      between central corneal thickness and the optic disc in an elderly population: the Bri-
      dlington Eye Assessment Project. Eye (Lond). 2009 Jan;23(1):56-62.

[60] Mokbel TH et al. Correlation of central corneal thickness and optic nerve head topog-
      raphy in patients with primary open-angle glaucoma. Oman J Ophthalmol. (2010)

[61] Cankaya AB et al. Relationship between central corneal thickness and parameters of
      optic nerve head topography in healthy subjects. Eur J Ophthalmol. (2008)

[62] Lesk MR et al. Relationship between central corneal thickness and changes of optic
      nerve head topography and blood flow after intraocular pressure reduction in open-
      angle glaucoma and ocular hypertension. Arch Ophthalmol. (2006)

[63] Insull E, Nicholas S, Ang GS, Poostchi A, Chan K, Wells A.Optic disc area and corre-
      lation with central corneal thickness, corneal hysteresisand ocular pulse amplitude in
      glaucoma patients and controls. Clin Experiment Ophthalmol. 2010 Dec;38(9):839-44.

[64] Nemesure B, Wu SY, Hennis A, Leske MC. Factors related to the 4-year risk of high
      intraocular pressure: the Barbados Eye Studies. Barbados Eye Studies Group. Arch
      Ophthalmol. 2003 Jun;121(6):856-62.

[65] Nicolela MT, Soares AS, Carrillo MM, Chauhan BC, LeBlanc RP, Artes PH. Effect of
      moderate intraocular pressure changes on topographic measurements with confocal
      scanning laser tomography in patients with glaucoma. Arch Ophthalmol. 2006 May;
      124(5):633-40.

[66] Park HY, Jeon SH, Park CK. Enhanced depth imaging detects lamina cribrosa thick-
      ness differences in normal tension glaucoma and primary open-angle glaucoma.
      Ophthalmology. 2012 Jan;119(1):10-20.

[67] Braunsmann C, Hammer CM, Rheinlaender J, Kruse FE, Schäffer TE, Schlötzer-Schrehardt U. Evaluation of lamina cribrosa and peripapillary sclera stiffness in pseudoexfoliation and normal eyes by atomic force microscopy. Invest Ophthalmol Vis Sci. 2012 May 17;53(6):2960-7.

[68] Lee EJ, Kim TW, Weinreb RN, Suh MH, Kang M, Park KH, Kim SH, Kim DM. Three-dimensional evaluation of the lamina cribrosa using spectral-domain optical coherence tomography in glaucoma. Invest Ophthalmol Vis Sci. 2012 Jan 20;53(1):198-204.

[69] Akagi T, Hangai M, Takayama K, Nonaka A, Ooto S, Yoshimura N. In vivo imaging of lamina cribrosa pores by adaptive optics scanning laser ophthalmoscopy. Invest Ophthalmol Vis Sci. 2012 Jun 26;53(7):4111-9.

[70] Kiumehr S, Park SC, Dorairaj S, Teng CC, Tello C, Liebmann JM, Ritch R. In Vivo Evaluation of Focal Lamina Cribrosa Defects in Glaucoma. Arch Ophthalmol. 2012 Jan 9.

[71] Viestenz A, Martus P, Schlötzer-Schrehardt U, Langenbucher A, Mardin CY. Impact of prostaglandin-F(2alpha)-analogues and carbonic anhydrase inhibitors oncentral corneal thickness. A cross-sectional study on 403 eyes. Klin Monbl Augenheilkd. 2004 Sep;221(9):753-6.

[72] Arranz-Marquez E, Teus MA. Relation between axial length of the eye and hypotensive effect of latanoprost in primary open angle glaucoma. Br J Ophthalmol. 2004 May;88(5):635-7.

[73] Arranz-Marquez E, Teus MA. Effect of previous argon laser trabeculoplasty on the ocular hypotensive action of latanoprost. Graefes Arch Clin Exp Ophthalmol. 2006 Sep;244(9):1073-6.

[74] Teus MA, Arranz-Marquez E, Lucea-Suescun P. Incidence of iris colour change in latanoprost treated eyes. Br J Ophthalmol. 2002 Oct;86(10):1085-8.

[75] Arranz-Marquez E, Teus MA. Effect of age on the development of a latanoprost-induced increase in iris pigmentation. Ophthalmology. 2007 Jul;114(7):1255-8.

[76] Arranz-Marquez E, Teus MA, Saornil MA, Mendez MC, Gil R. Analysis of irises with a latanoprost-induced change in iris color. Am J Ophthalmol. 2004 Oct;138(4):625-30.

[77] Viestenz A, Martus P, Schlötzer-Schrehardt U, Langenbucher A, Mardin CY. [Impact of prostaglandin-F(2alpha)-analogues and carbonic anhydrase inhibitors on central corneal thickness -- a cross-sectional study on 403 eyes]. Klin Monbl Augenheilkd. 2004 Sep;221(9):753-6.

[78] Harasymowycz PJ, Papamatheakis DG, Ennis M, Brady M, Gordon KD; Travoprost Central Corneal Thickness Study Group. Relationship between travoprost and central corneal thickness in ocular hypertension and open-angle glaucoma. Cornea. 2007 Jan;26(1):34-41.

[79] Sen E, Nalcacioglu P, Yazici A, Aksakal FN, Altinok A, Tuna T, Koklu G. Comparison of the effects of latanoprost and bimatoprost on central corneal thickness. J Glaucoma. 2008 Aug;17(5):398-402.

[80] Hatanaka M, Vessani RM, Elias IR, Morita C, Susanna R Jr. The effect of prostaglandin analogs and prostamide on central corneal thickness. J Ocul Pharmacol Ther. 2009 Feb;25(1):51-3.

[81] Zhong Y, Shen X, Yu J, Tan H, Cheng Y. The comparison of the effects of latanoprost, travoprost, and bimatoprost on central corneal thickness. Cornea. 2011 Aug;30(8): 861-4.

[82] Lopilly Park HY, Kim JH, Lee KM, Park CK. Effect of prostaglandin analogues on tear proteomics and expression of cytokines and matrix metalloproteinases in the conjunctiva and cornea. Exp Eye Res. 2012 Jan;94(1):13-21

[83] Weinreb RN, Toris CB, Gabelt BT, Lindsey JD, Kaufman PL. Effects of prostaglandins on the aqueous humor outflow pathways. Surv Ophthalmol. 2002 Aug;47 Suppl 1:S53-64.

[84] Crowston JG, Aihara M, Lindsey JD, Weinreb RN. Effect of latanoprost on outflow facility in the mouse. Invest Ophthalmol Vis Sci. 2004 Jul;45(7):2240-5.

[85] Amano S, Nakai Y, Ko A, Inoue K, Wakakura M. A case of keratoconus progression associated with the use of topical latanoprost. Jpn J Ophthalmol. 2008 Jul-Aug;52(4): 334-6.

[86] Agarwal DR, Ehrlich JR, Shimmyo M, Radcliffe NM. The relationship between corneal hysteresis and the magnitude of intraocular pressure reduction with topical prostaglandin therapy. Br J Ophthalmol. 2012 Feb;96(2):254-7.

[87] Bergonzi C, Giani A, Blini M, Marchi S, Luccarelli S, Staurenghi G. Evaluation of prostaglandin analogue effects on corneal keratocyte density using scanning laser confocal microscopy. J Glaucoma. 2010 Dec;19(9):617-21.

[88] Bolívar G, Teus M, Arranz-Marquez E. Effect of acute increases of intraocular pressure on corneal pachymetry in eyes treated with travoprost: an animal study. Curr Eye Res. 2011 Nov;36(11):1014-9.

[89] Wirtitsch MG, Findl O, Heinzl H, Drexler W. Effect of dorzolamide hydrochloride on central corneal thickness in humans with cornea guttata. Arch Ophthalmol. 2007 Oct; 125(10):1345-50

[90] Ornek K, Gullu R, Ogurel T, Ergin A. Short-term effect of topical brinzolamide on human central corneal thickness. Eur J Ophthalmol. 2008 May-Jun;18(3):338-40.

[91] Teus MA, Bolívar G, Alió JL, Lipshitz I. Short-term effect of topical dorzolamide hydrochloride on intrastromal cornealpressure in rabbit corneas in vivo. Cornea. 2009 Feb;28(2):206-10.

[92] Bolívar G, Teus MA, Hernández-Verdejo JL. Short-term effect of topical brimonidine tartrate on intrastromal corneal pressure in rabbits. J Refract Surg. 2010 Jul;26(7): 533-5. Surg 201;26(7):533-535.

Chapter 4

Malignant Glaucoma

Marek Rękas and Karolina Krix-Jachym

Additional information is available at the end of the chapter

1. Introduction

Malignant glaucoma was described for the first time and named so by Albrecht von Graefe in 1869 [1]. It is characterized by normal or increased IOP *(intraocular pressure)* associated with axial shallowing of the entire anterior chamber in the presence of a patent peripheral iridotomy [2,3]. The pathology is based on the existence of a block for normal flow of aqueous humour, which results in the accumulation of aqueous at an improper location in the eyeball [4]. The proposed mechanism involves a misdirection of aqueous humour passing posteriorly into or behind the vitreous gel [5]. This is a dynamic process, and if untreated, causes loss of vision. Local hypotensive treatment does not cause normalization of IOP, and conventional glaucoma surgery proves to be ineffective [3].

1.1. Classification

Classification includes phakic, aphakic, and pseudophakic malignant glaucoma. Aphakic malignant glaucoma is the onset of symptoms after a cataract surgery or the persistence of symptoms after treatment of phakic malignant glaucoma through the cataract extraction [6]. "Non-phakic malignant glaucoma" is a general term used for both types: aphakic and pseudophakic malignant glaucoma [6]. The term *malignant-like glaucoma* was proposed for cases with a known cause of forward displacement of the lens along with the frontal surface of the vitreous body other than the "trapping" of humour inside of the vitreous body [7]. There also exists a classification of malignant glaucoma into that occurring after surgical intervention and without such intervention [8].

The not fully known etiology of the process creates difficulties in the standardization of nomenclature. Certain authors suggest that the malignant glaucoma group should exclude cases in which e.g. pupillary block or choroidal detachment has been stated [9]. Others believe that using this term to encompass a broader spectrum of eye diseases will create a better understanding of the pathophysiology and the relationship between pathologies with similar clinical pictures [4].

1.2. Occurrence

According to literature, malignant glaucoma develops in 2% to 4% of patients with a history of acute or chronic angle-closure glaucoma that have undergone filtration surgery [3]. In own material, consisting of a total of 1689 penetrating and non-penetrating operations, performed as glaucoma surgery alone or combined with cataracts, malignant glaucoma occurred in 1.3% of all eyes after surgery. After penetrating surgery this complication was noted in 2.3% of eyes. It was also observed after laser iridotomy [10], phacoemulsification of cataract [11], posterior capsulotomy using a Nd-YAG laser *(Neodymium-yttrium-aluminum-garnet laser)* [12], cyclophotocoagulation [13], after implantation of large-sized IOLs *(intraocular lens)* [14], after local application of miotics [15], after suturolysis [16], and even in eyes that did not undergo surgical procedures [17]. Cases of malignant glaucoma have also been described in eyes in which glaucoma had not been established earlier [11].

Malignant glaucoma occurs significantly more frequently after penetrating surgery than in the case of non-penetrating surgery, after just the glaucoma surgery than after treatment combined with phacoemulsification, as well as in eyes with narrow angle glaucoma. It was stated with greater frequency among women, which may be related to the lesser dimensions of the anterior segment of the eyeball in this group of patients [18]. This complication can take place at various times after the operation, sometimes immediately, and sometimes after one year has passed or even after a longer period of time [3].

2. Anatomical basis

It is considered that incorrect anatomical relationships lead to disruptions in the direction of aqueous humour flow [4,19]. The place of increased resistance may be located at the level of the iris-lens, ciliary-lens, iris-hyaloid, and ciliary-hyaloid block [4,20]. Structures that are particularly related to the development of malignant glaucoma and its clinical picture:

Sclera – a thick sclera may lead to partial stenosis of the vortex veins, impairing normal venous outflow and causing overfilling of the choroid [21], as stated in eyes with malignant glaucoma [22]. Opening of the anterior chamber during surgery, which causes lowering of IOP, together with possible movements of the irido-lenticular diaphragm can trigger a malignant glaucoma mechanism in such eyes.

Lens – the exciting cause for malignant glaucoma in many cases is a lens that is too large for the eye [23]. Disproportions between its volume and the volume of the entire eyeball can occur; furthermore, particular anatomical relationships between the anterior vitreous, ciliary processes, and the lens foster the occurrence of malignant glaucoma [4,19].

Choroid – the choroid has a lobular structure with a tendency for accumulation of blood and thickening when outflow is impaired. Secondary, ciliary body and iris rotate to the front in patients with malignant glaucoma [24], closing access to the filtration angle from the back.

Vitreous body – Slit-lamp examination of the vitreous may reveal optically clear areas within the vitreous body – reservoirs of aqueous humour trapped in its gel structure [3], which may be confirmed on ultrasound [25]. In aphakic eyes, the anterior surface of the vitreous body may directly adhere to the ciliary processes [3].

The anterior and posterior chambers and their relationship – total obliteration of the posterior chamber by the vitreous and a highly resistant hyaloid membrane may be observed in aphakic and pseudophakic eyes [26].

3. Predisposing factors

The anatomic and functional differences of predisposed eyes seem to be a significant factor for determining the occurrence of malignant glaucoma. The following predisposing factors have been described, among others: axial hyperopia [27], nanophthalmos [28], disorders of anatomical proportions in the anterior chamber [18].

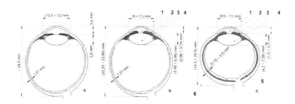

NORMAL EYE	RELATIVE ANTERIOR MICROPHTHALMOS (RAM)	NANOPHTHALMOS
	1 – Decreased corneal diameter	1 – Decreased corneal diameter
	2- Shallow anterior chamber	2- Shallow anterior chamber
	3 – Risk of the filtration angle closure	3 – Risk of the filtration angle closure
	4 – The lens takes up a disproportionately large percetnage of the volume of the eye	4 – The lens takes up a disproportionately large percetnage of the volume of the eye
		5 - Thickening of the choroido-scleral layer
		6 - Decreased axial length

Figure 1. Normal eye, relative anterior microphthalmos and nanophthalmos.

It is considered that malignant glaucoma is related to a special eye anatomy (small eye phenotype). Lynch et al. stated that it occurs more frequently in small eyes with an anatomically narrow iridocorneal angle [11]. Many nanophthalmic and RAM eyes have narrow angles with crowded structures in the anterior chambers. Typically, the lens is of normal or increased thickness, leading to a high lens:eye ratio and this crowding results in a shallow anterior segment that predisposes to angle-closure glaucoma [21]. In microphthalmos, due to small eye size, the increase in the size of the lens with age is critical, and a relative pupillary block forms with progressive shallowing of the central and circumferential anterior chamber, narrowing, and gradual angle closing [29]. However this is not the only angle closing mechanism in this pathology. Peripheral iridectomy, which eliminates pupillary block, does not prevent progressive overfilling of the choroidal bed, which may cause further angle closure. If the aqueous humour is directed to the vitreous cavity instead of the posterior chamber, symptoms of malignant glaucoma will occur [30]. Thus, in a genetically conditioned microphthalmos, glaucoma with a complex iris and ciliary block may be expected [20].

The occurrence of malignant glaucoma in the pathology that is the microphthalmos may not only be connected to abnormal anatomical relationships but also to incorrect histological structure of the sclera. The sclera in a microphthalmos is thicker relative to physiological conditions and its collagen fibers are more disorganized [31]. Trelstad et al. stated, that in a microphthalmos, collagen fibers of the intercellular substance in the connective tissue of the sclera have a normal thickness, but the collagen fibers are longer, less organized, and more interwoven [32]. Yue et al. stated that a greater heightened level of fibronectin, and speculated that a change in the glycosaminoglycan metabolism may influence the contraction of collagen fibers and lead to thickening of the sclera. The authors believe, that an incorrect glycosaminoglycan metabolism may cause a decrease in the elasticity of the sclera, which hampers normal development of the eye [33]. Based on known measurements of the thickness of the sclera, increased thickness of the tissues, including the retina, choroid, and sclera in echographic measurements was considered to be a value above 1.7 mm [34]. The increased thickness of the sclera in hyperopic eyes and its simultaneously lower surface area decrease transscleral protein transport, what, in consequence, causes choroidal expansion [22]. According to Quigley et al., a similar situation occurs in many eyes that do not achieve such small sizes, and malignant glaucoma can occur in eyes of correct sizes as well as in small eyes, but all cases would have dramatic choroidal expansion or vitreous flow abnormality [22]. In the case of a nanophthalmos, a tendency toward spontaneous or postoperative uveal effusion was also observed [21]. Quigley et al. observed that in eyes with extremely small sizes, displacement of the lens to the front occurs, caused by choroidal expansion [22]. Furthermore, the increased pressure in the vortex veins occurring in a microphthalmos as well as disrupted transscleral protein transport and increased oncotic pressure of the vitreous body may be linked to an increased risk of development of malignant glaucoma [21,22].

One of the more important factors predisposing the occurrence of malignant glaucoma is also partial or total closing of the filtration angle at the time of the surgery, especially if the malignant glaucoma occurred in the second eye [3]. However, IOP has no direct correlation to the risk of occurrence of malignant glaucoma. In Simmons's studies, the IOP level during the operation was not correlated with the probability of development of malignant glaucoma after surgery [3]. Moreover, it should be pointed out, that in the case of malignant glaucoma in one eye, the fellow eye exhibits a predisposition for occurrence of a malignant process [6].

4. Pathomechanism

The causes of malignant glaucoma are complex and there are several theories on the subject of factors that may have an influence on its development. As of now, the pathophysiological mechanism of malignant glaucoma is not yet fully understood. There is no certainty as to what structures or biochemical processes lead to the development of malignant glaucoma, and its cause seems to be conditioned by many factors.

An anterior rotation of the ciliary body processes, leading to ciliolenticular touch and ciliary block, has been suggested [25]. Forward displacement of a relatively large lens, which then blocks communication between the posterior and anterior chamber, as well as outlets from the eye, is the essential anatomical feature of malignant glaucoma [35]. Congestion of the uveal tract may play a part in pushing the lens into its forward position and holding it there [35]. In addition, in certain cases, the lens capsule and zonules may constitute a place of resistance for the flow of aqueous humour to the front [36]. The aqueous humour produced to the posterior chamber is directed to the back instead of to the anterior chamber [5], causing anterior displacement of the lens-iris diaphragm. Furthermore, swelling of the ciliary processes caused by inflammation or miotics can cause critical narrowing of an already anatomically narrow space between the lens equator and the ciliary body and relative block of forward aqueous flow [18]. Abnormal choroidal circulation may also lead to accumulation of blood and swelling of the ciliary processes. Moreover, Epstein and coauthors hypothesized that there is decreased permeability of the vitreous body or the anterior hyaloid to anterior flow of aqueous humour into the anterior chamber in malignant glaucoma [37].

Probably, there are eyes with predispositions for malignant glaucoma, in which there is a pathology of connective tissue related to a predominance of intercellular substance, mainly comprised of glycosaminoglycans. Glycosaminoglycans produced by fibroblasts of pathological connective tissue accumulate in the vitreous of such eyes with malignant glaucoma. Glycosaminoglycans, together with proteins gathered in the vitreous body because of impaired transscleral outflow, are responsible for the increase of oncotic pressure and accumulation of water. Moreover, high viscosity caused by mucopolysaccharides content makes the flow from the posterior to the anterior chamber more difficult. Glycosaminoglycans may also be a cause of iridocorneal angle damage.

The coexistence of anatomical and physiological predispositions and changes in IOP in the anterior chamber during surgery, activates a specific pump mechanism caused by movements of the lens-iris diaphragm, which may have an influence on the development of malignant glaucoma. The malignant process can have various dynamics with clinical manifestation occurring directly after surgery, when exciting factors cannot be compensated in the closed system of the eyeball. On the other hand, the occurrence of malignant glaucoma symptoms may be delayed if a relative equilibrium between the volume of the produced fluid and the outflow from the eyeball is reached

5. Objective symptoms

Myopic shift in refraction related to the anterior dislocation of the iris-lens diaphragm with secondary improvement of near vision [38].

Narrowing or shallowing of the circumferential and central part of the anterior chamber even if patent iridotomy or iridectomy is present. Shallowing of the anterior chamber is related to anterior dislocation of the iris-lens diaphragm [39,40] and iris-hyaloid diaphragm with coexistence of increased IOP [40]. Persistent symptoms of malignant glaucoma lead to the formation of intensified anterior adhesions due to the long-lasting shallowing of the anterior chamber [41].

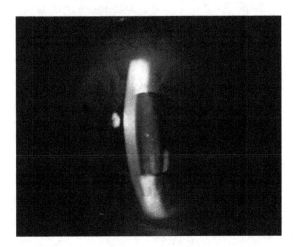

Figure 2. Axial shallowing of the anterior chamber in an eye with malignant glaucoma.

Increased IOP – intraocular pressure may increase slowly with simultaneously intensifying shallowing of the anterior chamber [42]. It is characteristic that in the presence of an active, well functioning filtering bleb, the increase in intraocular pressure can be moderate [43].

No decrease of IOP in response to conventional antiglaucoma treatment [4].

In many cases, a decrease of IOP or curing as a result of mydriatic-cycloplegic therapy [44].

Reaction to surgical treatment of the vitreous body [6].

6. Differential diagnosis

Glaucoma with pupillary block – pupillary block angle closure occurs when the posterior surface of the iris, in the pupillary margin, comes in contact with the lens. The increased pupillary block obstructs the flow of the aqueous humour from the posterior chamber to the anterior chamber, resulting in increased pressure in the posterior chamber and forward bowing of the peripheral iris. This closes the anterior chamber angle, obstructing the trabecular meshwork and the outflow channels with subsequent elevation of the IOP. Laser peripheral iridotomy is the treatment of choice [45] and should be performed in all cases of pupillary block glaucoma. In pupillary block, there should not exist axial shallowing of the anterior chamber (movement of the IOL toward the cornea). The anterior chamber usually remains deeper in the center than on its circumference, in contrast to malignant glaucoma, where axial chamber shallowing also occurs. If there is axial shallowing, then fluid has somehow moved posteriorly and the vitreous is acting to shallow the chamber [46].

Angle closure glaucoma – shallowing of the anterior chamber occurs symmetrically in both eyes. In the affected eye, the filtration angle is closed, there is a sudden increase in IOP, and microcystic edema of the cornea. Conjunctival injection and a medium size pupil may accompany these symptoms [47]. It occurs regardless of surgery and is caused by anatomical predisposition.

Choroidal effusion - a static condition which is observed independently of operation and has inflammatory (trauma and intraocular surgery, scleritis, following cryocoagulation and photocoagulation, chronic uveitis, Vogt-Koyanagi-Harada disease) or hydrostatic causes (hypotony and wound leak, dural arteriovenous fistula, abnormally thick sclera in nanophthalmos, possibly in emmetropic or myopic eyes or associated with Hunter's syndrome). Uveal effusion should not be considered to be a distinct clinical entity but rather a state characterized by abnormal amounts of fluid in the choroid resulting in thickening of the choroid, accumulation of fluid in the suprachoroidal space resulting in choroidal detachment, and in some cases, accumulation of fluid in the subretinal space, resulting in nonrhegmatogenous retinal detachment. IOP may be normal but is often reduced in uveal effusion secondary to inflammatory factors. An exception occurs in nanophthalmic uveal effusion wherein IOP is normal or frequently elevated and chronic angle closure glaucoma may develop [48].

Suprachoroidal hemorrhage – shallowing of the anterior chamber coexists with increased IOP, sudden pain, and the presence of a haemorrhagic, non-serous detachment of the choroid in biomicroscopic and ultrasonographic examination. It occurs most often within 1 week after surgery, rarely later [6]. Suprachoroidal hemorrhage may be caused by bleeding diathesis, anti-coagulants, paranasal sinusitis, or may occur spontaneously. Small suprachoroidal hemorrhages occurring during surgery are usually absorbed extemporaneously. Suprachoroidal hemorrhage may be also related to postoperative hypotony, and in the late postoperative period, may be connected to increased venous pressure or increased tension of the abdominal press.

7. Testing

Medical history – determination of predisposing factors and early statement of symptoms accompanying the occurrence of malignant glaucoma

Slit lamp examination – assessment of the depth of the anterior chamber shows that there is axial (central and peripheral) shallowing of the anterior chamber and, unlike in pupil block, the iris is not typically bowed forwards, and anterior lens movement is noted. Patency of the iridotomy, if such exists, should be evaluated – if there is no iridotomy or the patency is in doubt, laser iridotomy can be performed or repeated to rule out pupil block, but it does not cause resolution of the condition. Seidel test should be performed to exclude filtering bleb leaking after filtration surgery. Biomicroscopy assessment of the posterior segment is necessary for the purpose of ruling out choroidal detachment or suprachoroidal hemorrhage

Tonometry – usually reveals increased IOP

Ultrasonography – conducted for the purpose of determining the axial length of the eyeball (which tends to be shorter than normal) and to determine the position and size of the ciliary body and its processes [25]. Moreover, information on the thickness of the choroid may be obtained through ultrasonographic examination

Ultrabiomicroscopy (UBM) – this test gives images of the iris, the intraocular lens and ciliary body as well as their relative positions before and after the occurrence of malignant glaucoma. The rotation of the ciliary body to the front and shallowing of the anterior chamber may be subject to normalization after tearing of the anterior hyaloid [24]. This test enables visualization of the structures of the anterior segment, although the capability of conducting tests in the early postoperative period is limited due to the immersion technique

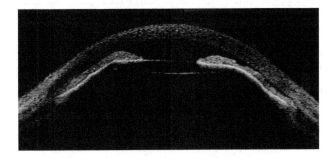

Figure 3. OCT of the anterior segment in malignant glaucoma – shallowing of the anterior chamber, peripheral iridocorneal touch, forward shift of the IOL.

Anterior segment OCT *(optical coherence tomography)* – a non-invasive high resolution technique that can be used for the purpose of objective imaging of the iridocorneal angle structure as well as for qualitiative and quantitative assessment. Parameters such as: AOD – *anterior chamber opening distance*, ACA – *anterior chamber angle* have been adapted from ultrasound biomicroscopy for the OCT method. Measurements of scleral thickness, CCT – *central corneal thickness*, and central depth of the anterior chamber during an episode of malignant glaucoma can also be conducted. Marked displacement of the structures of the anterior segment, peripheral irido-corneal touch, and forward shift of the lens may be noted Examination may reveal a decreased anterior chamber angle with extreme shallowing of the anterior chamber depth during the acute malignant glaucoma phase and an increase of ACA and AOD quantitative values after effective treatment of this condition. It is helpful to objectively evaluate the structures of the anterior chamber or to monitor changes in the anterior segment after surgery. Since the presence of corneal oedema is an indication of prompt surgical intervention it can be used to assess this parameter in a non-contact fashion [40].

8. Treatment

8.1. Conservative treatment

The goal of conservative treatment is to decrease the production of aqueous humour and shrink the vitreous while simultaneously decreasing resistance in the path of aqueous humour flow to the anterior chamber through applied cycloplegia.

The active mechanism of the drugs used in the treatment of malignant glaucoma is as follows:

Mydriatics – cycloplegics – paralysis of the ciliary muscle, widening of the ciliary processes ring, tightening of the zonule apparatus, backwards movement of the lens.

Osmotically active agents – increase of blood osmolality causing movement of water from the eyeball in the direction of hyperosmotic plasma, which results in a decrease of the hydration of the vitreous body and makes it possible to retract the iris-lens diaphragm and deepen the anterior chamber.

β-blockers – suppression of aqueous humour production, as a result of which the volume of humour directed towards the vitreous is reduced.

Carbonic anhydrase inhibitors – reduction of secretion of aqueous humour by inhibiting carbonic anhydrase activity in the epithelium of the ciliary body.

Corticosteroids – by limiting inflammation, they reduce edema in the area of the ciliary body and help to minimize inflammatory adhesions of the lens or vitreous body with the ciliary body [20].

According to data from the literature, approximately 50% of patients react to medical therapy [3]. In the work of Debrouwere et al., however, the percentage of recurrences after conservative treatment of patients with malignant glaucoma was equal to 100%, despite an initially good response to such therapy [49]. Also, in own experience, a lack of success in reversing the pathogenic mechanism by means of conservative treatment in malignant glaucoma concerns the great majority of cases. In own material, reactions to conservative treatment were observed in 5 eyes with malignant glaucoma out of 22 of those tested [22.7%), however, ultimately, a surgical procedure was necessary in three of them due to the recurrence of typical symptoms and no control over IOP. Permanent improvement after pharmacological treatment was achieved in only 2 eyes [9.1%). The observations of other authors also confirm transient effectiveness of medical therapy during the initial period [11,42]. Even if IOP control is achieved as a result of such treatment, long-term cycloplegia is necessary to maintain this effect in many eyes [25]. In some cases, when medications are discontinued or changed, tendencies of recurrence of malignant glaucoma symptoms are observed [50]. Therefore, medical treatment is thought to be of temporary effect and is used until definite treatment with laser iridotomy, posterior capsulotomy and hyaloidotomy is performed. The currently valid regimen for conservative treatment includes locally applied: atropine, phenylephrine, β-blockers, acetazolamide, and generally administered 50% glicerol solution in oral doses and intravenously administered mannitol. Locally applied corticosteroids play the role of limiting the accompanying inflammatory process. If improvement has been achieved, the dosage of hyperosmotic agents can be decreased, followed by carbonic anhydrase inhibitors, however treatment with mydriatic-cycloplegic agents should be continued [3]. The following treatment schedule can also be applied: mannitol 2 g per kg intravenously once or twice a day, acetazolamide 250 mg tid, and locally: 1% Tropicamide qid, Cosopt (dorzolamide hydrochloride-timolol maleate ophthalmic solution) bid, 0.1 % Dexamethasone phosphate tid. This regimen is usually successful until laser treatment is performed.

8.2. Surgical treatment

8.2.1. Laser treatment

Laser therapy is usually used together with conservative treatment and should be performed as early as possible because postponement of this therapy may lead to increased IOP with injury to the optic nerve and loss of visual field as a consequence, flattening of the anterior chamber, corneal-lens touch, and corneal decompensation. This method of management can also be used after malignant glaucoma surgery, and then can serve to sustain or restore the effects of the operation. The main limitation of laser techniques – excluding transscleral cyclophotocoagulation with a diode laser – is their dependency on corneal transparency. Topical glycerol may lead to temporary clearance of corneal edema and make the procedure viable.

In cases of suspected malignant glaucoma, pupillary block should be eliminated as a possible contributory element to the shallow anterior chamber by assessing the size and patency of iridotomy, when present, or by the creation of a patent iridotomy, if necessary [51]. Surgeons may prefer to use the Nd-YAG laser alone or argon laser pre-treatment followed by the Nd-YAG laser. With an Nd-YAG laser energy of 2-5 mJ, 1-3 pulses per burst are usually used.

Currently, as the treatment of choice in aphakic and pseudophakic eyes, several laser effects are used in combination: laser iridotomy with anterior hyaloidotomy and posterior capsulotomy, all through the same location. In this case, a positive effect of laser therapy is the creation of direct communication between the vitreous, the posterior chamber, and the anterior chamber, and such a procedure can restore normal dynamics of aqueous humour flow in malignant glaucoma [52]. If needed, it may be applied in more than one location.

Capsulotomy is usually performed using an energy of 1 to 4 mJ per pulse. The energy and pulses may be increased gradually according to the thickness of the capsule until an opening is achieved. 5-15 bursts with an energy of 1-3 mJ through iridotomy or iridectomy are usually effective in achieving communication. An immediate effect of such a procedure is often observed in the form of deepening of the anterior chamber. If there is no access to the iridectomy, communication can be achieved through the lens capsule in a pseudophakic eye using an energy of 1 mJ near the edge of the IOL. Such a procedure may be preceded by decompressing the vitreous chamber by puncturing it with a 25 gauge needle through pars plana. The above scheme may be repeated. The magnitude and patency of communication between the anterior and posterior segments of the eye are decisive to the distribution of pressure between the anterior and posterior segment of the eyeball. Recurrences may occur even when communication is present but is not effective enough to decrease the force shifting the iridolenticular diaphragm forward. In the case of difficult access to the circumferential part of the lens capsule in the area of iridectomy, the effect of deepening of the anterior chamber is to be achieved by creating a capsulotomy within the pupil or outside the edges of the artificial lens, after which a capsulotomy in the area of the iridectomy that is as large as possible should be created.

The goal of Nd-YAG laser hyaloidotomy, in turn, is to tear the anterior hyaloid face, as a result of which the depth of the anterior chamber is normalized [24]. Epstein and others treated aphakic and pseudophakic eyes with an energy of 3 to 11 mJ delivered to the anterior hyaloid face [53]. This treatment can be conducted through surgical iridectomies or laser iridotomies, often in many places. It is carried out centrally, to the back of the lens capsule, or in combination with capsulotomy in pseudophakic patients [46].

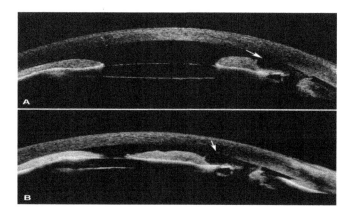

Figure 4. Anterior segment OCT in eye with malignant glaucoma – complication after Nd-Yag laser capsulotomy with hyaloidotomy - hyaloid gets across the iridotomy into the anterior chamber (white arrow); note shallow anterior chamber, forward movement of the IOL and iridocorneal touch at considerable area.

Transscleral cyclophotocoagulation is a procedure with different applications. The laser beam causes ablation of the ciliary body, which causes reduction of aqueous humour secretion. Energy absorption by melanine leads to thermal coagulation and destruction of the pigment epithelium and accompanying vessels. Deep coagulative necrosis of the pigment epithelium, pathological reconstruction of collagen fibers in the stroma, and intravascular coagulation in the blood vessels of the ciliary body take place [43]. Significant complications include postoperative inflammation, pain, cystoid macular edema, and phthisis. Thus, indications for cyclophotocoagulation are generally limited to patients whose glaucoma has been resistant to medical and surgical therapies, with no potential for improvement in visual acuity.

8.2.2. Surgical treatment

The indication for surgical intervention is a lack of effectiveness of conservative and laser treatment [11,36]. An operative procedure should not be conducted too late due to the development of complications resulting from the persistence of the malignant process.

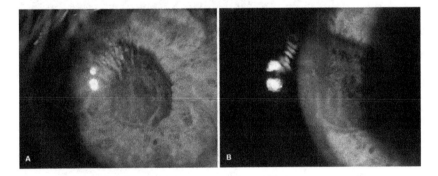

Figure 5. A,B: Advanced stage of malignant glaucoma - shallow anterior chamber, corneal oedema and posterior synechiae in pseudophakic eye.

Currently used methods of surgical treatment were introduced when the role of the pathology of the anterior segment and the vitreous body in the pathogenesis of the malignant process were discovered. As of now, surgical intervention in malignant glaucoma is directed towards lowering IOP, achieving correct anatomical relationships between the vitreous body, lens, and ciliary body, and additionally enabling correct flow of aqueous humour from the posterior segment to the anterior chamber of the eye. Achievement of communication seems to be necessary, because the disruption of aqueous humour flow in malignant glaucoma can last even after PPV [54]. The concept of such a procedure is based on the observation of regression of the symptoms of malignant glaucoma in the case of direct communication between the vitreous cavity and anterior chamber being ensured [25]. The iridectomy may be performed using Vannas scissors or a vitrectomy tip, whereas the posterior capsulotomy and hyaloidotomy may be done with a vitrectomy tip. The anterior chamber may be reformed with air. All of these procedures should be performed in one setting through the same location. Additionally synechiolysis may be performed if the iridocorneal angle is completely closed using a spatula or a viscoelastic agent. The performance of all three steps will usually result in complete resolution of the condition. Pars plana vitrectomy is reserved for cases that did not respond to the procedure above, and in any case, it should be combined with opening of the anterior hyaloid face. Thus, in refractory malignant glaucoma, partial PPV should be performed and supplemented by procedures making it possible to achieve communication between the anterior chamber and the vitreous cavity. Achievement of correct flow and equalization of pressure between the posterior and anterior segment of the eyeball is decisive for the effectiveness of the surgery. Partial PPV should be conducted conservatively, preferably using trocars and a 25 gauge vitrectome. Communication between the anterior chamber and vitreous cavity may be achieved by cutting out the lens capsule using a vitrectome or puncturing it through the cornea with a needle, alternatively by cutting the anterior and posterior capsules with cystotome from the side of the anterior chamber within iridectomy.

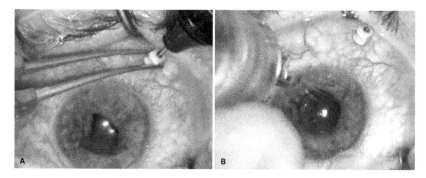

Figure 6. Combined partial pars plana vitrectomy with capsulotomy communicating anterior chamber and vitreous cavity in surgical treatment of malignant glaucoma: A. The trocar is inserted through pars plana 3.5 mm posteriorly to the corneal limbus before PPV. B. Achieving communication between the anterior chamber and vitreous cavity using a vitrectome.

9. Prognosis

Malignant glaucoma remains a difficult clinical problem that results in irreversible blindness if treatment is delayed and not adequate. The surgeon should be aware preoperatively of eyes at risk and observe them closely during follow-up visits. Early recognition is the most important step to prevent irreversible loss of vision. The prognosis depends on the duration and the severity of the malignant glaucoma attack. In patients with glaucoma in its early stage, the prognosis can be good if the attack is discontinued and IOP is well controlled. The problem is that malignant glaucoma is often resistant to conservative treatment, and laser procedures are not always effective as well. Partial pars plana vitrectomy combined with capsulotomy communicating the anterior chamber and vitreous cavity in such cases is an efficacious method of intervention when it comes to IOP control, postoperative BCVA, and reduction of the number of antiglaucoma medications. The prognosis after laser and surgica treatment depends on the occurence of complications after performed procedures. Complications after malignant glaucoma surgery observed in own material included: increased IOP during the early post-operative period (above 21 mmHg) [5%], inflammatory effusion [5%], hyphema [10%], occurrence of posterior adhesions [5%], no effectiveness of filtration surgery preceding the occurrence of malignant glaucoma [55%], macular edema [10%], and retinal detachment [5%]. Recurrence of malignant glaucoma with the full range of symptoms was observed in 15% of eyes subjected to surgery. In the case of post-operative shallowing of the anterior chamber, it is possible to conduct a capsulotomy through iridectomy, and the use of an Nd-YAG laser for this purpose is a safe and effective method in most cases.

10. Summary and conclusions

The condition continues to be one of the most difficult types of secondary glaucoma to manage. The diagnosis, definition, pathomechanism, and procedure in the case of malignant glaucoma still give rise to controversy. The currently applied treatment has the goal of unburdening the anterior chamber during the early period of the malignant process and to create communication between the anterior chamber and the vitreous. This is the result of the assumption, that in the case of a lack of communication through the iridotomy, recurrence of the malignant process can be expected after vitrectomy. New modifications of surgical procedure may increase operative effectiveness and improve the long-term results of applied procedures.

Author details

Marek Rękas and Karolina Krix-Jachym

Ophthalmology Department, Military Institute of Medicine, Warsaw, Poland

References

[1] Von Graefe A. Beitrage zur pathologie und terapie des glaucoms. Arch Ophthalmol 1869; 15:108-252.

[2] Muqit MMK, Menage MJ. Malignant glaucoma after phacoemulsification: treatment with diode laser cyclophotocoagulation. J Cataract Refract Surg 2007; 33(1):130-132.

[3] Simmons RJ. Malignant glaucoma. Brit. J. Ophthal. 1972; 56:263-272.

[4] Luntz MH, Rosenblatt M. Malignant glaucoma. Surv Ophthalmol 1987; 32:73-93.

[5]   Shaffer RN. The role of vitreous detachment in aphakic and malignant glaucoma. Trans. Am. Acad. Ophthalmol. Otolaryngol. 1954; 58:217-31.

[6]   Cyrlin MN. Malignant glaucoma. In: Albert DM, Jakobiec FA, editors. Principles and practice of ophthalmology. Philadelphia: W. B. Saunders, 1994:1520-1528.

[7]   Levene R. Malignant glaucoma: Proposed definition and classification. In Shields MB, Pollack I, Kolker A: Perspectives in glaucoma. Transactions of the First Scientific Meeting of the American Glaucoma Society. Thorofare, NJ, Slack, 1988:243-350.

[8]   Boke W, Teichmann KD, Junge W. Experience with ciliary block („malignant") glaucoma. Klin Monatsbl Augenheilkd 1980; 177:407

[9]   Simmons RJ, Dallow LR. Primary Angle Closure Glaucoma, in Duane TD (ed): Clinical Ophthalmology, Philadelphia, Harper and Row, Vol 3, Chap 53, 27-31, 1983.

[10] Brooks AMV, Harper CA, Gillies WE. Occurrence of malignant glaucoma after laser iridotomy. Br J Ophthalmol 1989; 73: 617-620.

[11] Lynch MG, Brown RH, Michels RG, Pollack IP, Stark WJ: Surgical vitrectomy for pseudophakic malignant glaucoma. Am J Ophthalmol. 1986; 102:149-153.

[12] Mastropasqua L, Ciancaglini M, Carpineto P, Lobefalo L, Gallenga PE. Aqueous misdirection syndrome: a complication of YAG posterior capsulotomy. J Cataract Refract Surg 1994; 20: 563-565.

[13] Azuara-Blanco A, Dua HS. Malignant glaucoma after diode laser cyclophotocoagulation. Am J Ophthalmol 1999; 127:467-469.

[14] Reed JE, Thomas JV, Lytle RA, Simmons RJ. Malignant glaucoma induced by an intraocular lens. Ophthalmic Surg 1990; 21:177-180.

[15] Rieser JC, Schwartz B. Miotic-induced malignant glaucoma. Arch Ophthalmol 1972;87:706-12

[16] DiSclafani M, Liebmann JM, Ritch R. Malignant glaucoma following argon laser release of scleral flap sutures after trabeculectomy. Am J Ophthalmol 1989;108:597-598.

[17] Schwartz AL, Anderson DR. "Malignant glaucoma" in an eye with no antecedent operation or miotics. Arch Ophthalmol 1975; 93:379-381.

[18] Razeghinejad MR, Amini H, Esfandiari H. Lesser anterior chamber dimensions in women may be a predisposing factor for malignant glaucoma. Medical Hypotheses 2005; 64:572-574

[19] Lois N, Wong D, Groenewald C. New surgical approach in the management of pseudophakic malignant glaucoma. Ophthalmology 2001; 108:780-783

[20] Weiss DI, Shaffer RN. Ciliary block (malignant) glaucoma. Trans Am Acad Ophthalmol Otolaryngol. 1972; 76:450-461

[21] Faucher A, Hasanee K, Rootman DS. Phacoemulsification and intraocular lens implantation in nanophthalmic eyes. Report of a medium-size series. J Cataract Refract Surg 2002; 28:837-842

[22] Quigley HA, Friedman DS, Congdon NG. Possible mechanisms of primary angle-closure and malignant glaucoma. J Glaucoma 2003; 12(2):167-180

[23] Birge H. Malignant glaucoma. Trans Am Ophthalmol Soc. 1956;54:311-328.

[24] Tello C, Chi T, Shepps G, Liebmann J, Ritch R. Ultrasound biomicroscopy in pseudophakic malignant glaucoma. Ophthalmology 1993; 100(9):1330-1334.

[25] Ruben S, Tsai J, Hitchings R. Malignant glaucoma and its management. Brit. J. Ophthal. 1997; 81:163-167

[26] Melanad S, Ashkenazi I, Blumental M. Nd-Yag laser hyaloidotomy for malignant glaucoma following one-piece 7 mm intraocular lens implantation. Br J Ophthalmol 1991, 75(8):501-503

[27] Sharma A, Sii F, Shah P, Kirkby GR. Vitrectomy-phacoemulsification-vitrectomy for the management of aqueous misdirection syndromes in phakic eyes. Ophthalmology 2006; 113:1968-1973

[28] Preetha R, Goel P, Patel N, Agarwal S, Agarwal A, Agarwal J, Agarwal T, Agarwal A. Clear lens extraction with intraocular lens implantation for hyperopia. J Cataract Refract Surg 2003; 29:895-899

[29] Simmons R. Nanophthalmos: diagnosis and treatment. In: Epstein D., ed. Chandler and Grant's glaucoma, Philadelphia: Lea & Febiger; 1986: 251-259.

[30] Steinert R. F. Cataract Surgery Third Edition, Chapter 33 – Nanophthalmos, relative anterior microphthalmos, and axial hyperopia. Elsevier Health Sciences, 2009.

[31] Epstein L. The malignant glaucoma syndromes. Chandler & Grant's Glaucoma 4th ed. Baltimore 1997; 285-292

[32] Trelstad RL, Silbermann NN, Brockhurst RJ: Nanophthalmic sclera. Ultrastructural, Histochemical, and Biochemical Observations. Arch Ophthalmol 1982; 100:1935-1938

[33] Yue BYJT, Duvall J, Goldberg MF, Puck A, Tso MO, Sugar J. Nanophthalmic sclera; morphologic and tissue culture studiem. Ophtalmology 1986; 93:534-541

[34] Wu W, Dawson DG, Sugar A, Elner SG, Meyer KA, McKey JB, Moroi SE: Cataract surgery in patients with nanophthalmos: Results and complications. J Cataract Refract Surg 2004; 30: 584-590

[35] Chandler PA. Malignant glaucoma. Trans Am Ophthalmol Soc 1950,48:128-143

[36] Harbour JW., Rubsamen PE, Palmberg P. Pars plana vitrectomy in the management of phakic and pseudophakic malignant glaucoma. Arch Ophthalmol. 1996;114:1073-1078.

[37] Epstein DL, Hashimoto JM, Anderson PJ, Grant WM. Experimental perfusions through the anterior and vitreous chambers with possible relationships to malignant glaucoma. Am J Ophthalmol. 1979; 88:1078-1086.

[38] Shahid H, Salmon JF. Malignant glaucoma: A review of the modern litereature. J Ophthalmol. 2012;2012:852659.

[39] Byrnes GA, Leen MM, Wong TP, Benson WE. Vitrectomy for ciliary block (malignant) glaucoma. Ophthalmology 1995; 102: 1308-11.

[40] Wribelauer C, Karandish A, Haberle K, Pham DT. Optical coherence tomography in malignant glaucoma following filtration surgery. Br J Ophthalmol 2003; 87(8):952-5.

[41] Tsai YY, T Sengs H. Combined trabeculectomy and vitrectomy for pseudophakic malignant glaucoma and extensive peripheral anterior synechia-induced secondary glaucoma. J Cataract Refract Surg 2004;30(3):715-7

[42] Greenfield D.S., Tello C., Budenz D. L., Liebmann J. M., Ritch R. Aqueous misdirection after hlaucoma drainage device implantation. Ophthalmology 1999; 106: 1035-1040

[43] Spaeth GL. Chirurgia okulistyczna. Rozdz. 39. Pooperacyjne spłycanie komory przedniej. Urban & Partner. 2006: 418-419.

[44] Chandler PA, Grant WM. Mydriatic-cycloplegic treatment in malignant glaucoma. Arch Ophthalmol 1962;68:353-359.

[45] Kanamoto T, Mishima HK. Angle closure glaucomas. In: Tombran-Tink J, Barnstable CJ, Bruce Shields M: Mechanisms of the glaucomas, Humana Press, 2008.

[46] Epstain DL. Pseudophakic malignant glaucoma – is it really pseudo-malignant? Am J Ophthalmol 1987; 103(2):231-233

[47] Kunimoto DY, Kanitkar KD, Makar MS. Podręcznik okulistyki. Lippincott Williams & Wilkins. Warszawa, 2007.

[48] Brockhurst RJ. Uveal effusion. In: Albert DM, Jakobiec FA, editors. Principles and practice of ophthalmology. Philadelphia: W. B. Saunders, 1994:1520-1528.

[49] Debrouwere V, Stalmans P, Van Calster J, Spileers W, Zeyen T, Stalmans I. Outcomes of different management options for malignant glaucoma: a retrospective study. Graefes Arch Clin Exp Ophthalmol. 2011; 08:20.

[50] Trope GE, Pavlin CJ, Bau A, Baumal CR, Foster FS. Malignant Glaucoma. Clinical and Ultrasound Biomicroscopic Features. Ophthalmology 1994; 101(6):1030-1035.

[51] Liebmann JM, Weinreb RN, Ritch R. Angle-closure glaucoma associated with occult annular ciliary body detachment. Arch Ophthalmol. 1998 Jun; 116(6):731-735

[52] Francis B, Wong R, Mincler DS. Slit-lamp needle revision for aqueous misdirection after trabeculectomy. J Glaucoma 2002; 11(3):183-188

[53] Epstein DL, Steinert RF, Puliafito CA: Neodymium:YAG laser therapy to the anterior hyaloid in aphakic malignant (ciliovitreal block) glaucoma. Am J Ophthalmol 98:137, 1984

[54] Francis BA, Babel D. Malignant glaucoma (aqueous misdirection) after pars plana vitrectomy. Ophthalmology 2000; 107:1220-1222

Chapter 5

Clinical Research Progress of Glaucomatocyclitic Crisis

He-Zheng Zhou, Qian Ye, Jian-Guo Wu,
Wen-Shan Jiang, Feng Chang, Yan-Ping Song,
Qing Ding and Wen-Qiang Zhang

Additional information is available at the end of the chapter

1. Introduction

1.1. Definition

Glaucomatocyclitic crisis was initially described in detail by Posner and Schlossman in 1948, so it was also called Posner – Schlossman syndrome (PSS). PSS is a special form of anterior uveitis with glaucoma, mainly seen in young adults, characterized by non-granulomatous iridocyclitis with significant elevation of intraocular pressure. In most cases, the disease took a form of acute, recurrent and monocular onset. [1, 2]

1.2. Morbidity

This disease is often seen in people aged from 20 to 50, and rarely in people above 60 years old. 5% or less of PSS cases were reported in people above 60 years old [3]. The disease is rare in Western countries, it was reported that 19 in one million people have suffered from PSS in Fenland [4]. As PSS is a kind of disease attacks intermittently,It is difficult to diagnose PSS in intermittent period for the lack of diagnostic signs and investigate the morbidity with epidemiology methods.We used the full text VIP Chinese literature retrieval system and Medeline retrieval system to find PSS reports from 1975 to 2011 in both English and Chinese literature and divided into review, case, experimental study and clinical report four categories,then analysed the regional distribution of the authors and cases (Chinese reports were divided into the Yangtze river and the other, English reports were divided into Asia and the other).

Chose the report which contained the most number of cases if there were more than two from the same author. Statistical results shows that 1262 cases were reported by 33 chinese clinical reports in which 991 cases reported by 20 reports from the area near the Yangtze river,and 271 cases reported by 13 reports from the other area. 211 cases were reported by 16 English clinical reports in which 144 cases reported by 7 reports from the asia area and 67 cases reported by 9 reports from the other area. The results above suggest that there are much more literature and cases related to PSS in the area near the Yangtze river and infer that the prevalence of PSS in that area may be higher.

Literature types	Region	Review	Case	Experimental research	Clinical report	Aggregate
Chinese	Near the Yangtze river basin	0	11	1	20	32
	Other areas	2	11	0	13	26
English	Asia	2	0	2	7	11
	Other areas	3	12	0	9	24
Aggregate		7	34	3	49	93(total)

Table 1. The regional distribution of the authors

1.3. Possible etiology

1. Many factors were considered to be related to the onset of PSS, such as allergy, fatigue, mental fatigue, mental stress, decreased body resistance, infection, hypothalamic disorders, autonomic dysfunction, abnormal reactions of ciliary vascular and nervous system and abnormal development in angle of anterior chamber.[1]

2. Recent research had confirmed that concentration of prostaglandins,(PGs) in the anterior chamber aqueous increased obviously in the PSS cases, especially that of PGE. [5]

3. Infection by herpes virus.

The conclusion that PSS was caused by herpes simplex virus (HKS) was reported by Yainamotos in 1995, and was confirmed by many following researches. A recent report showed that antiviral treatment reduced the frequency of the outbreak of the disease. [6-7]

It was reported that aqueous humor of a binocular PSS case were collected after suffering from herpes viral keratitis for five months with anterior chamber paracentesis, then DNA of cytomegalovirus (CMV) and HKS were measured by means of quantitative polymerase chain reaction(PCR), the results showed CMV was positive but HKS was negative. It was speculated that CMV which belongs to herpes virus genera would also leads to PSS like as wise. It was considered that PSS is not a separate disease, but a kind of anterior uveitis relating to infections of herpes virus.

A study from Singapore showed that the CMV DNA of aqueous humor was positive for 24 of 104 anterior uveitis cases with monocular high IOP, in which 18 cases were PSS, 5 cases were Fuchs heterochromic iridocyclitis (FHI). [8]Another study showed CMV DNA was positive in 35 of 67 PSS cases (52.2%), 15 of 35 FHI cases (41.7%). Although the kerato-precipitates (KP) in

CMV DNA positive anterior uveitis cases was consider to be accompanied with endothelial halo,clinical difference was not so significant between CMV DNA positive and negative cases as less aqueous humorin sample and weak sensitivity of detection method. In 2008, aqueous analysis for CMV by PCR was performed in 103 eyes of 102 patients with presumed PSS or FHI at the Singapore National Eye Centre. Their records were reviewed for clinical features and human immunodeficiency virus (HIV) status of the CMV-positive patients. The main parameters were age, gender, maximum intraocular pressure, endothelial cell count, endo-thelial changes, PCR results, and presence of uveitic cataract and/or glaucoma. It was found that there was no clinically detectable differences between CMV-positive and negative presumed PSS eyes. CMV-positive presumed FHI patients are more likely to be male, older at diagnosis or have nodular endothelial lesions. [9]

4.   Helicobacter pylori infection.

It was reported in South Korean that there was a significant difference of the positive rate of helicobacter pylori serum antibody between cases with PSS (80%) and cases without PSS(56.2%). In another prospective study, 40 cases with PSS and 73 cases without PSS received serologic analysis for the presence of H. pylori infection by an enzyme-linked immunosorbent assay. Positive rate of serum anti-H. pylori IgG was compared between the two groups. It was proved that H. pylori infection occurred significantly more often in PSS patients. This study suggests that exposure to H. pylori infection is associated with PSS in Korea. [10]

1.4. Clinical features of typical cases [1, 2, 3, 11, 12, 13]

1.   In most cases, the disease always attacks the identical eye repeatedly, binocularly affected cases is not common;

PSS result in paroxysmal increase of IOP repeatedly,which reaches as high as 40 to 60 mmHg, and lasts for 1 to 14 days generally,1 month occasionally,2 months rarely, interval of onset is from months to 2 years;

2.   Symptoms are not obvious, just mild discomfort for most cases;

3.   Eyesight is normal generally, blurred when suffer from corneal edema at onset;

4.   Pupil becomes bigger slightly with normal reaction to light, and never adheres to lens;

5.   The KP of PSS appeared in a few days after or before the elevation of IOP with number of 1 to 25, took a form of hoar and suet-shaped and disappeared days to 1 month after the IOP returned normal , distributed mainly in the inferior part of the cornea or concealed in the trabecular meshwork. There were no or at most a few planktonic cells in aqueous while the flare was negative .There is no inflammatory cell in vitreous body (See Figure 1);

6.   The anterior chamber angle is open, no matter IOP is normal or elevated;

Visual field and fundus of most cases is normal generally, but a reversible expanding of vascular shadow may occur during an acute onset;

7. Coefficient of outflow facility (C value) descends in episodes and recovery as IOP in intermission; various stimulation tests for glaucoma are negative in intermission.

8. The forms of onset of PSS could be divided into three kinds: KP, high IOP and intermediate type, according to relationship between KP and IOP.

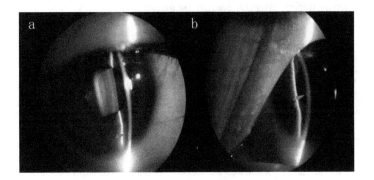

Figure 1. Anterior segment of a case with PSS in episodes. Arrows indicate the typical hoar and suet-shaped KP.

Typical case

The patient complained of her blurred vision two months ago, examination in other hospital showed: conjunctiva of her left eye wasn't congestive and the cornea was edematous mildly, IOP: 34/ 18(R/L) mmHg; there were some round lipid-like KP in the left cornea, aqueous flare (-). She came to our hospital on June 7, 2012, ophthalmologic examination: vision was 0.5/ 1.5(R/ L), best corrected vision of left eye was 1.2(-1.25DS), IOP: 18/ 13 (R/L) mmHg. Her right eye was normal, conjunctiva of her left eye wasn't congestive and there were five rounds lipid-like KP in the left cornea, binocular C/D was 0.4. Her KP faded away after the treatment of chloromethyl and pranopulin (three times a day) for three weeks. Examination of FFA, ICGA and Virus screening were normal on July 10.The measurement of her 24 hours IOP performed two weeks after she ceased the drugs was 20-14mmHg(R), 15-12 mmHg (L). The result of her visual field and the OCT for glaucoma was normal. She was diagnosed as PSS in left eye and suggested to be observed and treated timely.

1.5. Treatment of typical cases in episodes

1. Anti-inflammation: Corticosteroid drugs is needed in most cases, but it should not be used too long a time, so as not to cause the corticosteroid glaucoma.

It is a better select in some cases to apply non-steroidal anti-inflammatory drugs (NSAIDs) such as eye drops of pranoprofen, indomethacin and flufenamic acid.

Reducing IOP: Eye drops of epinephrine, timolol,or clonidine was needed singly or jointly for common patient, carbonic anhydrase inhibitor orally when the IOP is higher than 30mmHg and mannitol of intravenous drip when the IOP is higher than 40mmHg.

The antiviral treatment systemically or implanting long-acting agents maybe helpful to reduce the frequency of attack, but it has worrying and serious side effects and cost too much. [12]

2. The dispute and problems about prognosis

It was considered in the early years that PSS have a favorable prognosis without glaucomatous damage of optic disk and visual field, however, a number of authors have confirmed that part of the PSS cases suffered from glaucomatous damage similar to that in primary glaucoma patients in recent years. A lot of questions remained vague such as monocular or binocular, age of onset, the detailed features of its IOP and KP, the incidence and degree and relating factors of glaucomatous damage, especially the clinical approaches via which the damage occurred and disease complicated with PSS. These brought about to two undesirable consequences: first, PSS patients were misdiagnosed as primary glaucoma and received incorrect treatment even led to serious adverse consequences due to the lack of knowledge on the clinical characteristics of PSS.On the other hand, most cases of PSS combined with primary glaucoma patients especially these with primary angle-closed glaucoma were failed to be diagnosed correctly without delay, thus the best opportunity of treatment lost ; severe damage resulted in.

In order to solve the problems mentioned above, we have made a long-term systematic clinical study about PSS for more than 20 years persistently.

3. The main results of our clinical research

The main results of our clinical research included 4 fields as following: the clinical characteristics of PSS; the glaucomatous optic nerve damage in PSS patients; the clinical approach of optic nerve damage in PSS patients; other diseases concomitant with PSS.

3.1. Study on the clinical characteristics of the PSS

The research about clinical characteristics of the PSS included four aspects: clinical observation and analyzation of monocular primary open-angle glaucoma(POAG) and binocular PSS; clinical features of elderly PSS patients; characteristics and clinical value of the intraocular pressure and the C- value in PSS patients ; the characteristic of postural intraocular pressure change in PSS patients.

3.1.1. Clinical observation and analyzation of monocular primary open-angle glaucoma and binocular PSS

Background: As we knew, most of POAG patients are binocularly involved, while monocular attack is one of typical features of PSS. However, clinically suspected monocular POAG patient is not rare and binocular PSS cases are often reported. So following questions should be put forward based on the facts as follows [3, 11, 14]: Does monocular POAG really exist? What are the differences between monocular and binocularly involved PSS cases? Is there any relationship between the monocular POAG and binocular PSS?

Objects and methods

A long-term, systematic clinical observation and analysis were completed on 121 cases with tentative diagnosis of POAG (22 cases of monocular) and 126 cases of PSS (17 cases of which was binocular). (See figure2)

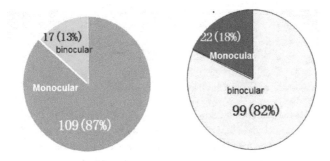

Figure 2. Distribution of monocular and binocular cases in PSS and POAG

Results

1. Glaucomatous visual field damage of monocular/ binocular PSS and binocular POAG

Analyzation of the clinical data of patients without doubt with the chi-square test showed: 1) The incidence of glaucomatous visual field damage in binocular PSS (15/16) was much higher than that in monocular cases(30/85), (X^2 =27.43, P<0.01). 2) The damage in 26 of 30 monocular cases were in early stage, while that in 9 of 15 binocular cases were in middle/ last stage, the difference was significant(X^2 =3.53, P<0.01).3) There is no significant difference in incidence and degree of glaucomatous visual field damage between binocular PSS and binocular POAG. (See Table 2)

Disease/ Visual field defect	Normal	Suspicious	Early stage	Moderate stage	Advanced stage	Absolute stage	Unknown	Total
Monocur PSS	55	7	26	1	2	1	17	109
Binoculus PSS	1	1	6	5	4	0	0	17
Binoculus POAG	4	7	22	8	39	7	12	99

Table 2. Visual field defect of monocular/ binocular PSS and binocular POAG

2. Visual field damage in binocular PSS

15 of 17 binocular PSS cases were confirmed with glaucomatous visual field damage, that was much more serious than in monocular cases; however, no remarkable difference was found between the course of disease in monocular and binocular cases. (See Figure3)

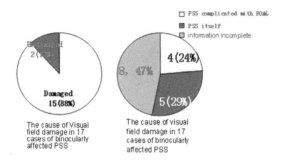

The cause of Visual field damage in 17 cases of binocularly affected PSS

The cause of visual field damage in 17 cases of binocularly affected PSS

Figure 3. Results of visual field examination and defect in binocular PSS.

The result suggests that the course of disease cannot explain the severity of visual field damage in binocular PSS. We speculate that binocular PSS may be more relevant to POAG essentially through the following two ways.First, the insufficiency in adjusting IOP result in combination with POAG in some cases; secondly, the weak resistance of optic nerve to high IOP make it ease for a cumulative effect of high intraocular pressure during attacks of pure PSS to bring about visual field damage.

3.   Results of clinical follow-up to monocular POAG

The results of clinical follow-up observation on the 22 cases with clinically suspected monocular POAG is as follows: 15 of the 22 cases were confirmed not to be POAG, 9 of them had been proved to be PSS. Although no definite diagnoses was made in the other 7 cases,but clinical manifestations contradictory with POAG were found in most cases, 3 of them were suspected of PSS.(See Figure4)

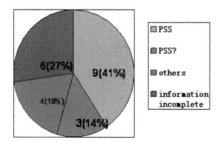

Figure 4. Results of clinical follow-up to monocular POAG.

The result suggests that the diagnosis of monocular POAG should be very careful, in addition to angle closure glaucoma and other secondary glaucoma, PSS which appears late or last transitorily should not be ignored. Close attention to slit lamp examination for KP and its relationship with IOP should be paid for such cases.

All in all, it cannot be stated too strongly: we should be very deliberative when making a diagnose of monocular POAG or binocular PSS, as half part of suspicious monocular POAG cases were confirmed with PSS after clinical follow-up, and there was a closer connection between binocular PSS and POAG. [15]

3.1.2. Clinical observation of aged PSS cases

Background: Among the cases of PSS, the 50s are rare; the 60s are seldom. What is the feature of the aged PSS cases?

Objects and methods: The clinical data of 14 cases aged above 50 with a definite diagnosis of PSS collected in the past 4 years were summarized and analyzed. Clinical data met all the requirements were obtained in 11cases. The cases aged from 50 to 73 years old, with an average of 61.4. 1 case had a course of the disease beyond 30 years, 4 beyond 10 years and 6 beyond 5 years.

Results: Visual acuity of more than half of the cases was inferior to 0.5, 9 of 11 cases had visual field damage that was of moderate or advanced stage in most cases.

Conclusion: The aged PSS cases had a longer course of the disease and much more frequent and serious visual function damage. [16, 17, 18]

3.1.3. The characteristics and clinical value of the intraocular pressure and the C- value in PSS cases

Background: It is generally acknowledged that IOP of the attacked eye increased and C- value of attack eye decreased in episodes, and both were normal in intermission. Individual author reported that the IOP of the affected eye was lower than that of the fellow one in part of cases, and C- value was higher. It was not confirmed that this phenomenon could be considered as the unique characteristic of PSS; and what clinical significance should it mean. [3, 19, 20]

Objective and methods: Binocular IOP measurement and tonography were done in 90 cases of PSS; According to the symptom, sign and results of examination for IOP, fundus, visual field, our cases were divided into 3 groups. Group A (typical type): with a normal optic disc, visual field and the diagnostic tests for glaucoma in intermission. Group B (development type): with a damaged optic disc and visual field; except for high intraocular pressure in episodes, binocular IOP and C values were normal. Group C (mixed type): with a damaged optic disc, visual field and abnormal results of binocular IOP, IOP diurnal variation and C value in both episodes and intermission. Another group case of primary glaucoma with a great fluctuation and difference in IOP level between his or her right and left eye was taken as the control group.

Results: IOP of PSS cases in group A and B increased in episodes, and were obviously higher than that of the fellow eye; C- value of them decreased and was lower. In intermission, binocular IOP and C- value turned normal, moreover, IOP of attacked eye was lower than that of the fellow one, and its C- value was higher. It means that binocular IOP and C- value in episodes and intermission were crossed-over.

Crossed-over phenomenon of binocular IOP and C- value had not appeared in the control group (primary glaucoma) as well as Group C (PSS combined with POAG). **Conclusion:** Such an inference could be deduced based on our results that Crossed-over phenomenon of IOP and C- value was one characteristic for pure PSS cases, it is conducive to distinguish pure PSS from primary glaucoma and PSS combined with POAG to observe this phenomenon. (See Figure5,6)

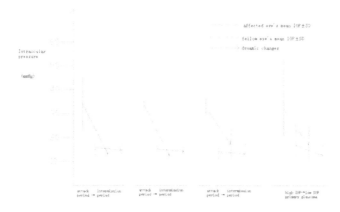

Figure 5. the difference of IOP and its dynamic changes between 3 PSS groups (A, B, C) and primary glaucoma.

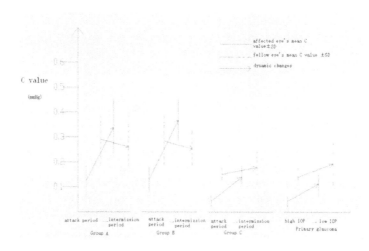

Figure 6. the difference of C- value and its dynamic changes between 3 PSS groups (A, B, C) and primary glaucoma.

3.1.4. The characteristics of postural IOP change in PSS cases

Background: It is well known that the recumbent IOP is higher than sedentary one in most of people; however, such an IOP change in PSS cases was not reported so far.

Objective: 83 cases of PSS with regular IOP change, 42 cases of POAG and 61 cases of PACG with a great wave in IOP level. [21]

Methods: IOP measurement was performed with a handheld applanation tonometer before and after laying for five and thirty minutes, and a tonography was finished 1~3 days before or after postural IOP measurement. (See Figure7)

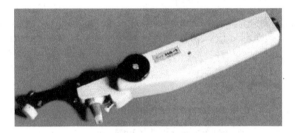

Figure 7. handheld applanation tonometer.

Results: 1) Recumbent IOP is much higher than sedentary one in cases of all groups, however, their rising degrees after laying were different.2) There was no significant difference of rising degrees after laying in three kinds of glaucoma when IOP was high; when the IOP turned normal, however, the rising degrees in POAG, PACG were much higher than in PSS. 3) When the sedentary IOP is higher than 24mmHg, the number of cases with recumbent IOP elevated more than 5mmHg in three kinds glaucoma wasn't different statistically; When the sedentary IOP is lower than 24mmHg, cases with recumbent IOP elevated more than 5mmHg were rare in PSS group, much less than that in the other two groups. 4) The IOP increment after laying in the attacked eye of PSS cases in episodes was much higher than that of the fellow eye and the both eye in intermission. 5) The IOP increment was related to C value significantly for POAG when IOP was high and normal, for PACG when IOP was normal only; But wasn't related for PSS no matter IOP was high or normal.

Conclusion: Measurement of postural IOP change is beneficial to diagnose suspicious glaucoma cases with a normal or slightly elevated IOP ,it maybe as valuable as tonography clinically but more convenient, comfort and safer than tonography, Complications such as corneal scratches were rarely seen in the measurement of postural IOP change

Discussion: Different pathogenesis of the three kinds of glaucoma accounts for the correlation between the IOP increment and C value in different conditions. PACG is caused by the closed anterior chamber angle, when the IOP is high, the increased IOP is related to C value significantly as the closed anterior chamber angle loses the ability to reduce IOP, however, the adjust ability recoverys as the anterior chamber angle open partly when the IOP is low. Degeneration of trabecular meshwork which result in more and more futile eduction function of aqueous humour was the primary mechanism for the increased IOP in POAG, so the IOP increment in POAG cases is related to C value significantly whenever the IOP is high or low as the adjust ability for IOP had been declining eventually. PSS is a secondary glaucoma for which the intermittent increased release of PGs maybe the primary mechanism. Increases PGs may expand the blood vessels and recedes eduction function of trabecular meshwork. On the contrary, the diluent PGs in remission promotes eduction function of aqueous humourm and turn IOP and C value to normal or even better. Therefore, there is no significant correlation between the IOP increment and C value no matter IOP was high or normal. [20, 22, 23]

3.2. The visual field damage in PSS cases

Although reports about that glaucomatous optical neural damage occurred in some cases of PSS were constantly released for past twenty years, we saw little of the systematic research aimed at the incidence, severity and probable relating facts of the damage. [3, 9]

3.2.1. Incidence and severity of the damage

Objective: To study the incidence and severity of the Visual field damage in PSS cases.

Methods: Visual field examinations at regular intervals with perimeter of Goldmann or Humphrey 750 type were completed in 145 cases of PSS followed up for 5 to 15 years and 166 cases of POAG observed meanwhile (as the control). [17]

Results: The prevalence of visual field damage in PSS and POAG was 35.43% and 93.42% (P<0.001), 72.11% of the field damage in PSS cases was of early or suspected stage, 78.92% of that in POAG cases was of middle or late stage(P<0.001), 10% of PSS cases suffered a field damage of middle or late stage, 2 became absolute blind and one case had developed into bullous keratitis at last.(See Figure8)

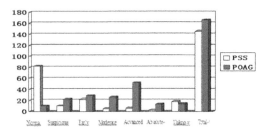

Figure 8. the stage distribution of visual field damage in PSS and POAG.

Conclusions: Even the visual field damage in cases of PSS was less and slighter than that in cases of POAG, It is necessary to treat PSS efficiently and timely, as recurrent attacks of PSS for long period would result in a sad outcome like POAG.

3.2.2. The characteristic of the visual field damage in PSS

Objective: To study the characteristic of the visual field damage in PSS.

Methods: Compare the visual field damage in glaucoma cases with higher and lower IOP (PSS belongs to that with higher IOP). [24]

Results: 1) The visual field damage in cases with lower IOP is less and slighter than that in cases with higher IOP. 2) Paracentral, arcuate and ring scotoma was more seen in cases with normal IOP, while constriction of visual field and nasal field were more common in cases with higher IOP. 3) Most of the visual field damages in cases with higher IOP comes from the periphery. (See Figure9)

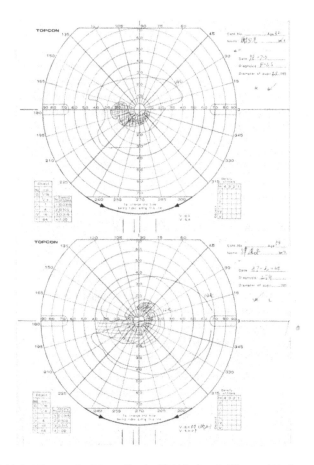

Figure 9. Visual field of a PSS case and a LTG case. The visual field damages in PSS case exist in the periphery area (A), on the contrary, those in glaucoma case with normal IOP exist in the centre area (B).

Conclusions: There are difference visual field defects between higher IOP patients and lower IOP patients.

3.2.3. Relating factors of the visual field damage in PSS

Objective: To study the relating factors of the visual field damage in PSS.

Methods: Analysis the clinical data of 145 PSS cases and 166 POAG cases for recent 15 years. Results about the incidence and severity of visual field damage in the two kinds of glaucoma had been showed above.

Results: 1) Compared with the undamaged group of PSS, the damaged cases were older and with longer course of the disease while there was no remarkable difference in the averaged IOP value during crisis. 2) There was a much higher risk for the visual field damage in binocular cases of PSS. Most of the cases of PSS reported were monocular affected, but later, there were reports about some binocularly affected cases. In our study, 15 of the 35 cases with definite damage were binocularly affected while only one of the 82 cases without damage was affected binocularly. It needs further study to determine whether there is different pathological mechanism for the monocular and binocularly involved cases of PSS. 3) IOP manifestation: although no great difference in the average IOP value during crisis was found between the two groups of PSS, the damage group showed a higher average IOP between crises and included much more cases with an abnormal diurnal and nocturnal variance of IOP or without the IOP crossed-over phenomenon than the undamaged group. These data indicated that the adjustment of IOP between crises was insufficient in those PSS patients with visual field damage. Loss of IOP crossed-over phenomenon meant that other than PSS there were some factors affecting the IOP. [25]

Conclusions: These data indicated that the harmful effect of the raised IOP during crises of PSS on the optic disc could be accumulated.

3.3. The clinical approach of optic nerve damage in Posner Schlossman syndrome

In recent years a number of authors have confirmed that glaucomatous optic nerve damage similar to that in primary glaucoma cases occurred in part of the PSS cases, but the clinical approach of the occurrence was not reported. Clinical data of cases with PSS during a period of 25 years in our hospital was collected and analyzed, and four clinical approaches via which the damage occurred in PSS cases were deduced.

3.3.1. Propose

To investigate the clinical approach of optic nerve damage in PSS.

3.3.2. Methods

208 cases with PSS during the recent 25 years collected in our hospital(male 124 cases, female 84 cases), from 9 to 71 years old, with an average of 39.56±12.80. Diagnosis standard for PSS

was basically accorded to clinical features described by Posner and Schlossman, except for the cases who suffered binocularly or had damage were contained in. [23, 26]

Research project of first diagnosis at the first attendance in our hospital

History, eyesight, intraocular pressure of episode and intermission, depth of anterior chamber, gonioscope or UBM, intraocular pressure during 24 hours in intermission without eyedrops more than five days, panretinalscope or OCT, FFA in episode of part cases, and so on.

Analytical methods

1. Analysis for damage

Standard: repeatable glaucomatous visual field damage and corresponding fundus performance

2. Stage division standard of glaucomatous visual field damage(see Table3)

Without defect	static visual field: no more than 2 spots with sensitivity reduces more than 5dB , no spot with sensitivity reduces more thandB; dynamic visual field: no nasal step and temporal more than 10 degrees, no significantly constriction of visual field (except for refractive interstitial lesions and retinopathy)
Early stage	paracentral scotoma, nasal step, , arcuate scotoma not linked with physiological blind spot
Moderate stage	arcuate scotoma linked with physiological blind spot, nasal hemianopsia,ring scotoma, constriction of visual field more than 30 degrees,
Advanced stage	tubular
Absolute stage	no light perception

Table 3. Stage division standard of glaucomatous visual field defect

3. Classification method

According to the results of comprehensive and dynamical analyzation to the clinical data of each cases and classification method shows as table 4, each case was discriminated for the clinical approach of optic nerve damage. [20,21,22,24,27,28]

	A Early stage	A Later stage	B Early stage	B Later stage	C Early stage	C Later stage	D Early stage	D Later stage
Age of onset	middle-aged and aged people		middle-aged and aged people		similar to POAG		middle-aged and aged people	
Family history of glaucoma	usually not		usually not		sometimes have		most have	
Monocular/	monocular		monocular		binocular or monocular		monocular KP, binocular high IOP	
Typical PSS course	positive	positive	positive	negative	Intermittent attack with KP		positive	negative
IOP Episodes Sick eye	rise	rise	rise	rise	higher	higher	rise	rise
IOP Episodes another eye	normal	normal	normal	normal	high	high	high*/ normal	high*/normal
IOP Intermission Sick eye	normal	normal	normal	rise	high	high	high*/ normal	high*/normal
IOP Intermission another eye	normal	normal	normal	normal	high	high	high*/ normal	high*/normal
Cross phenomenon of intraocular pressure	positive		positive	negative	negative	negative	positive */ negative	positive */ negative
Intraocular pressure of 24 hours in period of intermittent	normal	normal	normal	abnormal	abnormal	abnormal	abnormal */ normal	abnormal */ normal
Anterior chamber depth	normal	normal	normal	normal	normal	normal	A little shallow	Very shallow
Anterior chamber angle	medium width	medium width	medium width	medium width	medium width	medium width	Narrow II-III	Narrow III-IV

*When adhesive closure of the angle or damage of trabecular meshwork occurred.

Table 4. Classification method of the clinical approach for optic nerve damage in PSS

3.3.3. Results

1. Incidence and stage distribution of glaucomatous optic nerve damage

190 cases of 208 patients with PSS had a set of complete material. There were 71 cases (34.1%) with optic nerve damage, in which 12 cases (16.9%) regarded as suspicious damage, 59 cases (83.1%) regarded as definite damage.

Stage distribution of glaucomatous optic nerve damage was shown in Table 5:

Early stage	Moderate stage	Advanced stage	Absolute stage	Total
35	11	11	2	59
59.32%	18.64%	18.64%	3.39%	100%

Table 5. Stage distribution of glaucomatous optic nerve damage in 59 cases regarded as clear damage

2. The clinical approach of optic nerve damage

Four clinical approaches via which the damage occurred in PSS were deduced, they were represented as Type A, B, C and D.

Type A Cumulative effect of repeated episode of high intraocular pressure of pure PSS leads to visual field damage: 27 cases

Type B Recurrent attacks of PSS which results in secondary trabecular meshwork damage causes secondary open-angle glaucoma: 6 cases

Type C PSS combined with primary open-angle glaucoma: 19 cases

Type D PSS combined with primary closed-angle glaucoma: 7 cases

Composition of the clinical approach in 59 cases regarded as definite glaucomatous optic nerve damage was showed in Figure10.

3. Distribution of stage of visual field damage in different optic nerve damage approaches was showed in Table 6

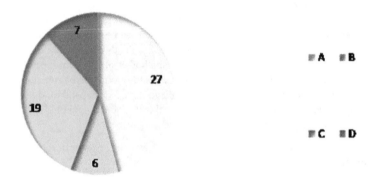

Figure 10. The distribution of clinical approach of optic nerve damage in PSS.

	Early stage	Moderate stage	Advanced stage	Absolute stage	Total
Type A	17	7	1	2	27
Type B	2	2	2	0	6
Type C	5	7	7	0	19
Type D	2	3	2	0	7

Table 6. Stage distribution of Visual field damage in different type of PSS patients

There is not significant difference in the stage distribution of visual field damage in different type of PSS patients. ($X2 = 6.904$, $P>0.05$).Make the early and moderate stage as one group, advanced and absolute stage as anothe group, Statistical result shows that there is significant difference in the stage distribution of visual field damage in different type of PSS patients.The incidence of early stage of glaucomatous visual field damage in Type A (63%) was higher.While 7 of 19 Type C cases were in advanced stage.

Conclusion: Most cases in type A suffered a early stage damage, and most in other types suffered a moderate or advanced stage damage, but there were 2 cases in type A who had gone to absolute stage.

3.3.4. Discussion

1.   The clinical approach of optic nerve damage in Posner-Schlossman syndrome.

In the past PSS was considered to be a self-limited disease and has a favorable prognosis,however, in recent years a number of authors have confirmed that part of the PSS cases suffered glaucomatous optic nerve damage similar to those in primary glaucoma cases, but the incidence, degree, related factors and clinical approach of the occurrence is unknown. This part focused on the clinical approach of optic nerve damage in Posner-Schlossman syndrome after aforementioned researches. Report about optic nerve damage caused by PSS combined with primary open-angle glaucoma is common; the other types were seldomly reported.Systematic research aimed at this question has never been seen so far at home and abroad. We determined the damage approach by analyzing each patient's clinical data dynamically and comprehensively according to the discrimination method established on the basis of relating literatures and the results of our long-term systematic study, and got the conclusion that there were four clinical approaches via which the damage occurred. Beyond all question, further researches, supplement and correct is necessary in this field, but the method and result of our study maybe a wind vane for the further researches.

2.   Clinical features and treatment principle for cases with damage from different clinical approach

3.3.4.1. Type A Cumulative effect of repeated episodes of high intraocular pressure of pure PSS leads to damage

Clinical features

Except for visual field damage, type A cases complied with the basic characteristics of typical PSS: monocular attacked; intermittently onset of high intraocular pressure with hoar and suet-shaped KP ;normal intraocular pressure(including 24 hours intraocular pressure)of the fellow eye in episode and the both eyes in intermission ; Crossed-over phenomenon and postures change of IOP; Normal anterior chamber depth; wide anterior chamber angle; Visual field change of vascular shadow usually appears in episode and recover in intermission at the initial in most cases, and true visual field damage is of mild and early stage usually , but loss of light perception can be seen in a few cases; the attack lasts a long time frequently in middle-aged and aged people for long course, also with higher IOP; heterochromia iridis occurred in later stage in some cases. (See Figure11) [20, 22, 29]

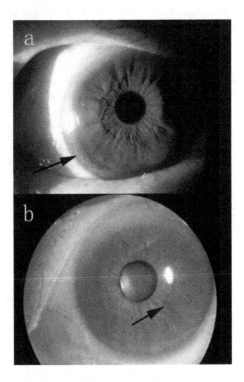

Figure 11. The iridis of a PSS patient. (A) is that of the normal eye (B) is that of the affected eye.

Treatment principle

Pay enough attention to treatment for each attack, in which the most important is controlling intraocular pressure timely and effectively. Surgery is necessary for the cases with excessive frequent attacks, heavy damage or obvious progress of his damage.

The surgery method and the time: glaucoma valve or EX-press glaucoma filtration device implantation maybe suit for cases with excessive frequent attack, high IOP but light inflammation (intermission or episodes); trabeculectomy could be selected for cases with low attack frequency, high IOP as well as severe inflammation (intermission only).

Typical cases

1) She visited our hospital and was diagnosed as glaucomatocyclitis crisis of left eye in other hospital six years ago. In the initial stage, she attacked once or twice per year with duration of 3~7 days for each attack and ceased spontaneously, then the frequency of attack increase

and the duration extended. This attack happened one month before this visits to our hospital and stop one week ago without use of any drug.

Examination at first visit: Vision 1.0(OU), IOP19.7mmHg(R), 12mmHg (L), anterior chambers of both eyes were not shallow, iris color was symmetrical, KP (-).

Fundus examination: C/D0.3(R) 0.6(L), there wasn't other abnormalities. She was diagnosed as secondary glaucoma of left eye. On September 13 (10 days after withdrawal), the 24 hours IOP of both eyes were measured: right eye: 14-18mmHg, left eye 12-14mmHg, Corneal thickness: right eye: 584μm, left eye: 575μm. She was diagnosed as "glaucomatocyclitis crisis in left eye."

Another onset lasted for more than 10 days, IOP of the left eye was 43mmHg, there was 2 hoar and suet--like KP and faded iris pigment in left eye. There were total seven attacks in oneyear, with the duration from 1 week to 20 days, during one of which the KP appeared 9 day after the occurrence. 24 hours IOP during this episode: right Eye: 14-19mmHg, left Eye: 23-29mmHg; iris depigmentation of her left eye exacerbated, no abnormal was found with fundus angiography. The recent onset occurred in September this year, the medication of hormone and pranopulin continued for 3 months, with another minor attack during that this period.

She made another visit to our hospital one year later. It was found that the iris of her left eye appeared a typical "rain dozen sand samples", meanwhile, there were two off-white round medium-sized lipid-like KP.and she was diagnosed as "left eye glaucomatocyclitic crisis with heterochromatic iris." Since then, the attack occurred more frequently, with frequency of 1 to 2 times per month, the visual field damage exacerbated. She was hospitalized in our department, and the surgery of glaucoma valve implantation was performed. Postoperative intraocular pressure: 19mmHg for her right eye and 6mmHg for her left eye:, visual acuity:: 1.0 left eye (with pink hole) for her both eye, and the syndrome did not attack postoperation. (Clinical data please see Figure 12)

2) He was hospitalized in our hospital for the reason of "intermittent pain of left eye for 25 years, decrease of vision for 20 years, blind for 1 year".

Since 25 years ago, the patient got intermittent episodes of pain and blurred vision with his left eye, which occurred 1 to 2 times per month with the duration of 3to 5 days, and can be self-cured. In many hospitals he was diagnosed as "glaucomatocyclitic crisis" and treated with irregular medication. The occurrence becomes more frequently in the recent 10 years, and the duration longer, and the vision recessions gradually.

In the intermittent period, he was hospitalized for systematic examination. Visual acuity was 1.0 for his right eye and no light perception for his left eye. All the results of IOP, tonography, 24 hours IOP measurement and other tests during the intermittent period were normal for his both eyes.

The result of the medical examination at this hospitalization showed as fellowing: his right eye had a corrected visual acuity of 1.0, IOP 14mmHg, C/D 0.4, wide anterior chamber angle; his

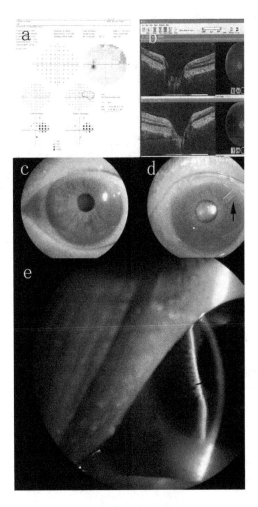

Figure 12. Clinical data of a cases suffered from PSS with glaucomatous optic nerve damage combined with heterochromia iris (Clinical number 488368). Visual field (A) and Optical Coherence Tomography (B) indicate glaucoma damages; Anterio segment of normal right eye (C) and left eye (D), arrow shows heterochromia iris and KP in the attacked eye (E).

left eye had no photoreception, intraocular pressure 56mmHg, C / D1.0, width of N1 ~ N3 for the anterior chamber angle with some small limited adhesions; corneal edema, a dozen of round lipid-like KP.

Without any treatment, the IOP of his fell to 14mmHg within one week. All results of examinations including 24 hours IOP measurement, drinking water experiment, darkroom prone test for his right eye were normal. Laboratory results of systemic body check were normal.

His left eye still had attacks of PSS after he left hospital and each attack could be self-cured. IOP and 24-hour IOP during the intermittent period were measured to be normal, and his left eye had an IOP lower than that of his right eye, a typical IOP cross phenomenon appeared every time. Three years later, the fundus and visual field of his right eye kept normal. (Clinical data see Figure 13)

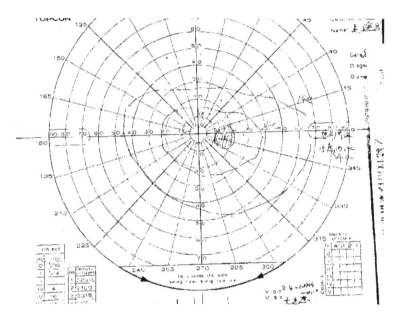

Figure 13. Visual field of the right eye of patient (Clinical number 241163). PSS results in blind of his left eye, but the visual field of his right eye without PSS is normal.

3.3.4.2. Type B secondary open-angle glaucoma from secondary damage to trabecular meshwork by recurrent attacks of PSS

Clinical features

Type B cases complied with the basic characteristics (above mentioned) of typical PSS in early stage. These characteristics lost eventually as the damage to trabecular meshwork gradually accelerated, the attack takes place more frequently and lasts a longer and longer time with a higher and higher IOP, and serious visual field damage developed at last. [30, 31] However, the fundus, visual field, IOP in intermittent and episode of the fellow eye maintained normal. Patients of this type usually had a long course of the disease with an order age.

Treatment principle

It is necessary to reduce IOP with drugs according to extent and characteristics of elevated IOP and diminish inflammation with hormone of weak effect on elevating IOP for short time, for example, lotemax. PGA is useful and myotic is prohibitive. Surgery or other treatment (SLT, trabeculectom, glaucoma valve or EX-press implantation) should be taken into account according to the IOP level controlled by drugs in intermittent and the situation of visual field damage.

Typical case

He was diagnosed as "left eye PSS" with the complain of vision decline associated with distending pain of his left eye in other hospitals five years ago.

The medical records of other hospitals showed: IOP and other relating examinationgs of his right eye in episode and these in intermittent period of his both eyes was normal at the initial stage. The visual acuity decreased gradually, IOP fluctuated from 32 to 48 mmHg in recent years. He was hospitalized in our hospital three times, the results of clinical observation showed: IOP including 24 hours IOP in intermittent period, the fundus and visual field of his right eye appeared normal; while IOP of his left eye was high frequently and higher when PSS attacked, 24 hours IOP in intermittent period appeared abnormal including the highest IOP and IOP variation. The left eye was diagnosed as secondary open-angle glaucoma from secondary damage to trabecular meshwork by recurrent attacks of PSS, and then a trabeculectomy was performed on his left eye. Postoperative IOP of his left eye was from 12 to 10 mmHg in intermittent period, 20 to 31 mmHg in episodes, while his right eye kept normal in all ways. (Clinical data see Figure 14)

3.3.4.3. Type C PSS combined with primary open-angle glaucoma

Clinical features

Monocular/ binocular paroxysmal increased IOP with mild cyclitis; wide anterior chamber angle; binocular abnormal IOP and visual field damage; high average IOP; grate fluctuation of IOP level; absence of IOP cross phenomenon; PSS attacks at the same eye in most cases; at the two eyes alternately or at the same time in a few cases; visual field damage was serious, and more serious in the eye often attacked by PSS. [27, 32]

Treatment principle

Enough attention should be given to the treatment for cases of this type, whose incidence reached up to 31% as reported.

Drug treatment is similar to that of POAG, but in episode of PSS, corticosteroid is useful transitorily, while PGA and myotic is prohibitive. Indication of surgery is similar to that of POAG, but classical trabeculectomy should be performed in intermission, and the effect and safety of nonpenetrating trabeculectomy, implantation of Ahmed glaucoma valve or EX-PRESS Glaucoma Filtration Device has not been confirmed. Laser trabeculoplasty(ALT), Selective laser trabeculoplasty (SLT) or Pneumatic trabeculoplasty (PNT) should be adopted in intermission, however, there has not related report. [11, 33, 34, 35]

Typical cases

1) With complaints of discomfort and blurred vision of her left eye for more than 1 year, the patient was diagnosed as POAG in other hospital 10 days ago. Clinical date of that time

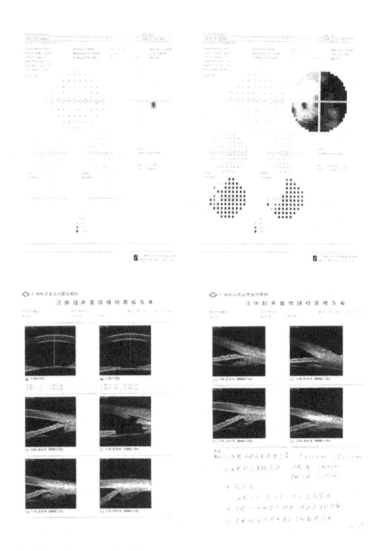

Figure 14. Clinical data of a patient suffered from PSS with glaucomatous optic nerve damage due to secondary open angle glaucoma (Clinical number 81304). Normal visual field in right eye (A) and advanced visual field defect in left eye (B); UBM shows the normal right eye and the affected left eye post-operation (C).

showed: KP (-), IOP16.3/42.7(R/L), and she was treated with Travoprost Eye Drops to her left eye and brimonidine and brinzolamide to the both eye. 1 week after treatment, her IOP turned to 36/17(R/L), the treatment had been changed to travoprost, brimonidine and brinzolamide for the both eye.

The results of examination in our hospital showed as follows: visual acuity R1.0 (-1.25DS), L0.05(-3.75DS), IOP17(OU); absence of conjunctiva hyperemia; cup/disc ratios 0.8 OD and0.9 OS,and inferior RNFLD(by OCT:) in the both eye; severe glaucomatous visual field damage in both eye.;extended latent time and descended amplitude on VEP; CCT:540/520 (R/L),corneal endothelium cells 1730/2747(R/L); center anterior chamber depth ≥3.0mm and open anterior chamber angle in every direction for the both eye by UBM. She was diagnosed as binocular POAG,and treated successively with travatan, alphagan and brinzolamide to binoculus, but her IOP was not controlled well. Thus, a trabeculectomy was performed the left eye.Two weeks after the operation, the filtration bubble turned fibrosis,and IOP increased. By 3 times of pin-delamination with 5- fluorouracil and eyeball massage, IOP was controlled on 12 to 14 mmHg. Her right eye was treated with travatan, carteolol hydrochloride and brimonidine, IOP was controlled from 12 to 14 mmHg.She was discharged from hospital.

Four months later, the right eye appeared 5 small rounds and mutton-fat like KP, IOP increased to 19mmHg. A week late, KP played down, IOP descended to 12 mmHg. A month later; KP appeared again, IOP increased to 37, after treatment in hospital for a week, the IOP decreased to 12 mmHg. She was diagnosed as POAG combined with PSS. Two months later PSS of her right attacked again, IOP increased to 44 mmHg; visual field damage has progressed remarkably. FFA showed optic atrophy without any other abnormal. She was hospitalized again,and a implantation of Ahmed valve to her right eye was done on the next day. During the operation, the valve appeard out of control; we dealt it well with removable restraint line processing; the IOP and anterior chamber stability was controlled. 2 month after the operation, the IOP increased to 22 mmHg because of the draining disc was packaged. By pin-delamination and eyeball massage, IOP was controlled near to 20mmHg. Carteolol hydrochloride was added and the IOP was controlled well in intermittent, but PSS attacked frequently and the IOP was out of control during episode. she was hospitalized once more and the right eye was treated with no-penetrating glaucoma surgery. 1 month after operation, the IOP was controlled well, binocular IOP was 10mmHg. 2 month after operation, PSS attacked her right eye again, IOP increased to 20 mmHg. This attack faded a week late and IOP of her both maintained 14mmHg below until now. (Clinical data please see Figure 15)

2) She was diagnosed as POAG in other hospitals because of intermittent attacks of distending pain and gradually aggravated blurred vision to her right eye for six years. The left eye has the same symptoms slighter than that of her right eye.

When she was examined in our hospital the results showed as follow: visual acuity: R 0.4, L 0.2; IOP: R 50mmHg and L 17mmHg; anterior chamber angle NI~NII in every direction; The optic cup depressed and enlarged. Argon laser trabeculoplasty was carried out after the diagnosis of POAG. But after that, the right eye relapsed frequently. One year later, the right eye relapsed again. There were three KP which were gray-white, round, and like mutton-fat in the right eye and a wreck of the keratic precipitate in the left eye. After a series of relating examinations such as visual activity, IOP, fundus, visual field, gonioscopy, she was diagnosed as PSS.

Seven years later, the patient attended to our clinic because the same symptoms attacked frequently in recent years and her vision became worse and worse. Attacks appeared as binocular

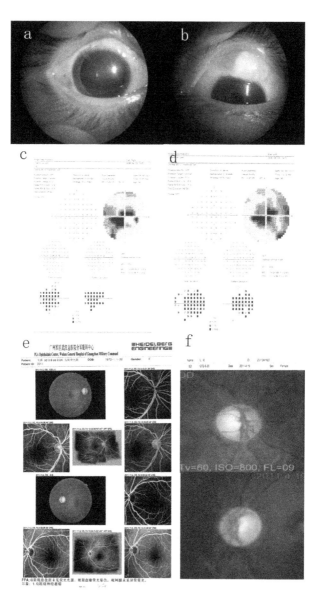

Figure 15. Clinical data of patient suffered from PSS(right eye) with glaucomatous optic nerve damage combined with POAG(both eye). The right eye is treated with Ahmed valve implantation surgery (A), the left eye is treated with normal trabeculectomy (B), visual fields of right eye (C) and left eye (D) show typical glaucoma damages, the fundus angiography indicates no vascular disorder except of optic atrophy (E) and the optic cups of right eye and left eye are non-symmetrical (F).

high IOP with binocular KP or binocular high IOP with monocular KP in different time. Clinical data on this visit showed :visual acuity: R 0.2, L 0.15;there has not obvious keratic precipitates in the right eye, but the left eye has one mutton-fat like keratic precipitate; the ratio of C/D was about 0.9; IOP was R 28 mmHg and L 31 mmHg; the visual field has deteriorated over the last few years; 24-hour IOP measurement during the intermittent period showed that IOP of the right eye was from 21 to35mmHg and 23 to 36mmHg for her left eye.Thus,PSS combined with POAG was proved to be the last diagnosis. Her visual acuity and visual field were in a stable condition under regular treatment with carteolol Hydrochloride 2% and brimonidine tartrate as well as anti-inflammatory drug when PSS attacks. (Clinical data see Figure 16)

3.3.4.4. Type D PSS combined with primary closed-angle glaucoma

Research status

Except for our data, there had been only two individual reports about PSS combined with PCAG in China and none in abroad. Cases of PSS combined with PCAG at home are much more than those in abroad due to the higher incidence of PCAG as well as PSS at home. In 2004 we reported 6 cases and completed a systematic clinical analysis. It was often reminded by many ophthalmologists that cases of PSS had be mistaken as AACG, but enough attention had not been paid to this type of PSS. [18, 28, 36, 37, 38]

Clinical features

There is a typical history of PSS attack with binocular shallow anterior chamber and narrow or closed anterior chamber angle. PSS hardly attacked synchronously with PACG, the anterior chamber angle is open in episodes of PSS. Type D cases complied with the basic characteristics of typical PSS in early stage: binocular IOP is normal in intermission; with cross phenomenon of IOP; however, when PACG became more advanced, although the IOP of the PSS attacked eye was much higher than that of the unattacked eye in the episode of PSS, binocular IOP turned higher than normal even in intermittent of PSS without obvious cross phenomenon. Most cases were diagnosed as PACG previously, PSS appeared after the treatment for PACG had been completed and the anterior chamber angle been opened, a few cases were typical PSS with narrow anterior chamber angle when they were young; PACG appeared as anterior chamber angle became narrower and narrower with age. Most of the cases of this type were elder with a longer course of PSS and a more advanced visual field damage.

Diagnosis standard

The first is that the anterior chamber angle is open when PSS is diagnosed at episode, either in the intermission of PACG or after PACG was treated with Laser/surgery/drug; the second is that the cases complied with the basic characteristics of typical PSS described by Posner-Schlossman. In our study, 2 cases was diagnosed as PSS at a younger age with binocular narrow anterior chamber angle (first was narrow II, narrow III-IV four years later), 5 cases was diagnosed as PSS after treatment of PACG(similar to the two cases reported at home). [28, 39]

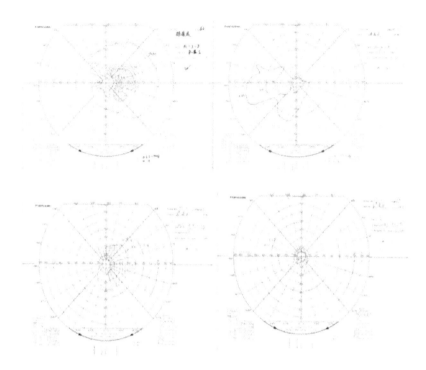

Figure 16. Visual field of patient (Clinical number: 232036) with binocular PSS combined binocular POAG. After drug treatment, the damages of binocular visual fields between1991 (A) and 1998 (B) has no significant advance.

Diagnostic gist

To find out PACG complicated with PSS as soon as possible, it is necessary to carry out a set of comprehensive and careful examinations relating to PACG in the intermission of PSS for PSS patients with factors as follows: the old-aged ,with a serious visual field damage, longer course of the disease, with a shallow anterior chamber or an narrow anterior chamber angle,and binocularly attacked.

When IOP appeared as repeated, intermittent and sudden elevation in a patient with PACG whose anterior chamber angle had been opened and the IOP been controlled well for a period after treatment by means of laser and/or surgery and/or drugs, it is very important to pay sufficient attention to the depth of the binocular anterior chamber and anterior chamber angle on the time the IOP is higher, and to make clinical follow-up observations for KP and its relationship with IOP, so as to ascertain whether PSS is the cause of elevating IOP, so that unnecessary surgery can be avoid.

Treatment principle

According to condition of PACG, laser and/or surgery and/or drugs may become options.

Laser treatment:

1. Indications of that for cases of PSS combined with PACG is similar to that PACG patients, except for that examination and treatment should be done in the intermission of PSS;

2. Curative effect on cases with typical cross phenomenon of IOP should be better;

3. The iris surrounding excision mouth by laser must be thoroughly penetrated and the hole should be big enough;

4. Corticosteroids and drugs for reducing IOP should be sufficient after laser operation;

5. It is import to pay attention to the treatment for PSS which continue to attack after laser therapy, and to the monitor of IOP and its dynamic change. Additional drug treatment even trabeculectomy should be adopted timely when necessary;[27]

It is necessary to prevent the attack of PACG in either episodes or intermission of PSS for these untreated PACG cases with the appropriate use of miosis drug.

Typical cases

1) He was diagnosed as "PSS" in our hospital because of pain and discomfort of his right eye,then he was diagnosed as " acute angle-closure glaucoma " in other hospital because of severe sore of his both eyes, and switched to our hospital after remission seven years later.

Examination revealed mutton-fat like KP in the right eye. His right eye was diagnosed as PSS combined with PACG with analysis by synthesis combining history and test results of IOP, fundus, visual field and anterior chamber angle. The right eye was treated with "glaucoma drainage surgery", and the left eye with "YAG laser iridectomy ".

IOP of his both appeared stable for six months after operation, then the right eye was attacked by PSS once again. This attack of PSS appeared as typical KP, open angle and slightly increased IOP. (Clinical data please see Figure 17)

2) The patient came to our clinicbecause of "Repeated intermittent attacks of eye pain and impaired vision for her left eye and right eye as well for more than 14 years". She was treated with YAG laser iridotomy in other hospital for PACG binocularly twice each.,Her left eye had been still attacked intermittently ever since.Clinical date from her medical record showed that KP and IOP rising appeared nearly simultaneously on each episode and the IOP turned persistently higher than normal even if in intermission since 2 years ago, and the drugs could not control the IOP well.

Examination at this time showed: Vision R 1.0, L 0.4; IOP R 14 mmHg and L 46 mmHg ;2 mutton-fat like KP in the left eye ; shallow anterior chamber and angle multiple adhesions in the both eyes; several trace of lasertherapy on iris of her both eye,the only panetrated hole on the right eye be covered with fibrous membrane, and that on the left eye be too small; cup/disc ratios R 0.4 and L 0.8.A diagnosis of "binocular PACG complicated with PSS in left eye" was established.A complementary lasertherapy was given to her right eye just at that moment; after this lasertherapy,her right had been kept well until now with only the help of 2% Carteolol Hydrochloride Eye Drops twice a day.3 weeks late, when this attack of PSS fade away, she was hospitalized in

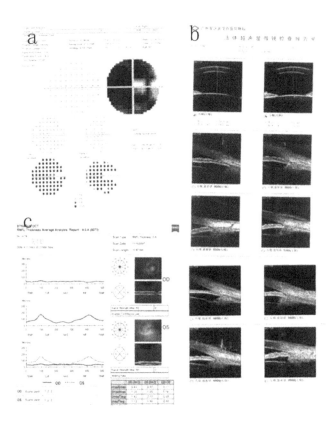

Figure 17. Typical clinical data of patient (Clinical number: 406013) with diagnosis of right PSS combined with binocular PACG and treatment with classical trabeculectomy. The visual field show advanced glaucoma damages(A), OCT (C) also shows retinal nerve fiber layer defect, UBM indicate binocular closed angle (B).

our hospital,and a trabeculectomy was performed on her left eye, and she was discharged 10 days after a IOP of 14mmHg.6 weeks after the operation, an attack of PSS occurred with a IOP of 32mmHg and lasted a week;such attack occurred once or twice a year after that with a maximal IOP of 25mmHg. The IOP in intermission had maintained near 15mmHg during the first 4 years, but the result of 24h IOP measurement showed 13~20mmHg in the right eye and 15~24mmHg in the left eye. Iris heterochromia appeared in the left eye. Such a therapeutic schedule was established and kept 3 years since then: 2% Carteolol Hydrochloride Eye Drops twice a day to the both eye in intermission of PSS; 2% Carteolol twice a day plus brimonidine 3 times a day with shortly use of Lotemax for the left eye during episode of PSS. IOP of the both eye maintained 15mmHg or below, and the visual field maintained stable in the 3 years.

Several attacks of PSS had been recorded with a IOP up to 40mmHg, and her visual field turned worsen, and "rain dozen sand -like" appearance in the iris of her left eye got more pronounced in the last 2 years. She was hospitalized once more, and another trabeculectomy was performed on the left eye near the first one, at the end of which the two filtering blebs(an original and a just manufactured) were merged into one. She was discharged with an IOP of 12mmHg; the left eye was no longer attacked after this trabeculectomy ,and the IOP kept stable.

(Clinical data see Figure 18)

4. Main points in diagnosis and treatment of complications of PSS

Other kinds of glaucoma which PSS concurred with or lead to were introduced before. PSS can also concur with or cause iris heterochromia, ischemic optic neuropathy, complicated cataract and other diseases, such as retinal detachment. Main points in diagnosis and treatment of these complications were briefly introduced as follows:

4.1. PSS combined with iris heterochromia

Typical cases

1) The patients came to our hospital because his left eye suffered from intermittent recurrent pain and blurred vision for more than one year. Intraday examinations showed: best corrected visual acuity is 1.0/ 0.6(R/L), IOP: 16.7/ 13.7(R/L) mmHg, FFA in both eyes are normal, optic cup in his left eye is expand. He was suspected of glaucoma. Intermittent recurrent pain and blurred vision kept to attack his left eye for more than half a year after then. These attacks usually ceased a few days late, with or without the help of 0.5% timolol eye drop and other drugs. During this period, the highest IOP record of his left eye was 35mmHg with a normal record of his right eye. The patient returned to our hospital one year later after stopping use of any drugs for two weeks. Ophthalmologic examination at this time showed: visual acuity 1.2 both eyes, IOP 17/15(R/L)mmHg, a lot of small lipid-like KP in the inferior of the left cornea, "rain dozen sand -like" appearance in the iris of his left eye, C/D rate 0.6/0.7(R/L),CCT 553/ 560(R/L). Results of his visual field and OCT showed in Figure below. UBM showed wide-angle in the both eyes. Fundus fluorescein angiography and contrast sensitivity revealed no special finds. 24 hours IOP measurements(2 weeks after KP disappeared): 13~16/ 12~15(R/L) mmHg. Diagnosis of "PSS complicated with iris heterochromia" for his left eye was confirmed than.He was asked to treat every onset of the disease in time with drugs dropping IOP as well as anti-inflammatory medicine. (Clinical data see Figure 19)

2) She was admitted to our hospital because her right eye suffered from repeated episodes of pain with blurred vision for more than nine years, and her vision decreased 3 months, with a primary diagnosis of "secondary glaucoma" for her right eye. A lot of intermittent recurrent pain and blurred vision had attacked her right eye from nine years ago, 2 or 3 times a year. Each attack lasted about one week, than resolved spontaneously. Three months ago her sense of vision went to recession. She felt that her right eye was attacked again recent days, so she can to our hospital. Ophthalmologic examination in this time showed: visual acuity: 0.15/ 1.0 (R/L), IOP: 43/12(R/L) mmHg, mist edema in her cornea of her right eye with a lot of fat-like

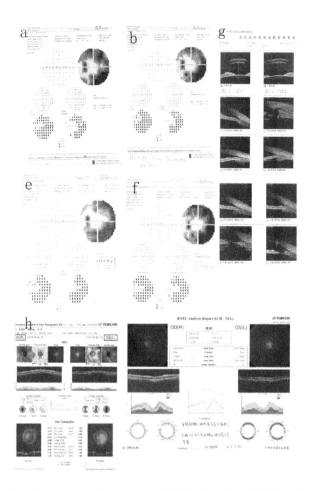

Figure 18. Typical clinical data of patient (Clinical number: 341555) suffered from left PSS combined with binocular closed-angle glaucoma. The visual fields of right eye(A) and left eye(B) become worse 4 years later(C) and (D), UBM indicate binocular aqueous humour outflow after the 1st trabeculectomy(E) and the OCT results show serious retinal nerve fiber layer defect in left eye (F).

KP, pale and"rain scatting beach-like" appearance in her left iris with a round pupil about 3mm in diameter, her optic disk appeared pale in color with a C/D 0.9, her anterior chamber is not shallow, ultrasound biomicroscopy (UBM) showed a wide angle in both eye. Her left eye showed no KP with a C/D less 0.3. Her systemic examination and routine inspection and examination showed no special finds. Treatment with drugs dropping IOP such as carteolol and brimonidine and even mannitol as well as anti-inflammatory medicine such as loteprednol kept about a week, KP significantly reduced but the intraocular pressure is still high. Operation

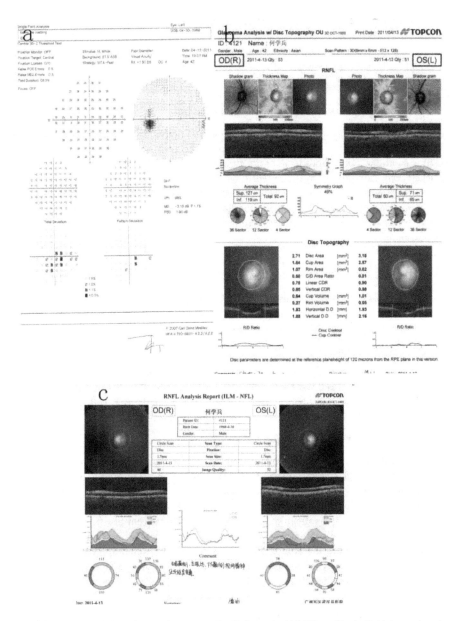

Figure 19. Typical clinical data of patient (ID: 11041302) with diagnosis of left PSS combined with iris heterochromia. Visual field of left eye show nasal defect(A), binocular OCT results indicate ocular cups expand(B)and (C)obvious retinal nerve fiber layer defect(C).

of Ahmed valve implantation was performed on her right eye two weeks larer. She was discharged a week postoperative with an IOP of 9mmHg in the operated eye. Her IOP was controlled well with fewer attacks of PSS and a stable visual field in the recent 3 years after the operation. (Clinical data see Figure 20)

Discussion

1.   Clinical performance of PSS complicated with iris heterochromia

4 cases of PSS complicated with iris heterochromia were reported [40]. They were 2 males and 2 females aged 35 to 45 years. In addition to typical PSS performance, the iris showed "rain scatting sand-like"appearance in all of the 4 patients. All of them are monocular repeatedly attacked at the same eye. Each attack kept 3 to 7 days with a significantly increased IOP up to 30.00 ~ 60.00mnHg and a few of fat-like KP, than relieve itself or extinct with the help of medication. Intraocular pressure (including 24 hours intraocular pressure) in intermittent period appeared normal after discontinuation of all medication with a typical crossed-over phenomenon.

2.   Key-points in the differential diagnosis between PSS complicated with iris heterochromatic and FHI (Fuchs heterochromic iridocyclitis).

The two diseases are different clinically in the following five aspects: the attacked eye and sex of patients, manifestation of intraocular pressure, character of KP, appearance of the Lens and Glaucomatous damage of optic nerve and visual field.

The attacked eye and sex of patients

Most of PSS cases were monocular affected, a few of cases was binocularly attacked but alternately between left and right eye, extremely rare cases was both eye attacked simultaneously. Male patient is more than female in PSS. FH is generally believed that no gender differences, more than 90% of the cases was monocularly effected.

Manifestation of intraocular pressure

The IOP in patients of PSS with iris heterochromatic appeared as an intermittent and abruptly rising when the attack comes with the appearance of typical KP in pure PSS patients. IOP elevation in patients of PSS with iris heterochromatic usually lasted 3 ~ 10days, and then turned to subside spontaneously with the disappearance of the KP after this period, it is also sensitive to drugs dropping IOP and anti- inflammatory medicine. On the contrary, IOP of patient with FH appeared normal in the initial stage for a long time, after that,elevated in part of the cases gradually; however, once the intraocular pressure elevated, it often appeared persistently higher, although there maybe some fluctuations. The elevated IOP and KP in patient with FH had no characteristic of intermittent, were difficult to be controlled and poorly responded to corticosteroids therapy.

IOP in patients with PSS complicated with iris heterochromatic kept the characteristic of crossed-over, that is, the IOP of the attacked eye was higher than that of contra lateral eye during the episode but lower(3 ~ 5mmHg) than the other eye between attacks. IOP in patients with Fuchs syndrome had no such characteristic, once elevated; it is always higher if untreated.

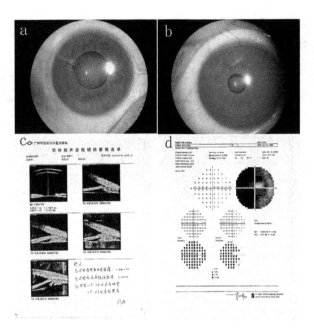

Figure 20. Typical clinical data of patient (Clinical number: 437614) with diagnosis of right PSS combined iris disorder. The right eye is after Ahmed implantation and arrow indicate iris heterochromia (A), the left eye is normal (B). UBM indicate a wild angle in right eye(C), but the visual field show serious damages in right eye (D).

KP

The KP in patient with PSS complicated with iris heterochromia appeared only in a short period during the attack in most cases. This KP is of following characteristics: small round suet-like, medium sized, isolated, with no pigment in initial stage, mainly located in the lower part of the cornea, usually disappeared naturally within a few days after or before IOP reduction. On the contrary, KP in patients with Fuchs syndrome has different characteristics as following: persistence for very long time even always in most cases, white transparent small dot or star-like coexisting with pigmented KP, diffuse distribution in the cornea, sometimes connected each other with fibrous filaments, poor response to corticosteroids therapy. (Clinical data see Figure 21)

Lens situation

Fuchs syndrome complicated with cataract is common at later stage; however the complicated cataract is uncommon in the PSS cases with iris heterochromia.

Glaucomatous retinal and visual damage

Glaucomatous damage in PSS cases appeared later and to a lesser extent, however that of FHI cases occur earlier and quicker.

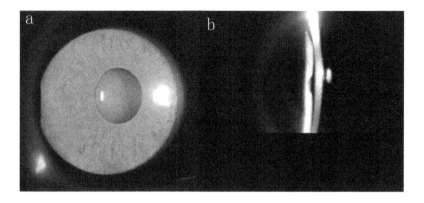

Figure 21. Heterochromatic iris and KP in FHI. There is a typical iris such as "rain dozen sand -like" (A) arrow shows a lot of star-like pigmented KPs (B).

4.2. PSS combined with ischemic optic neuropathy

Typical cases

The patients came to our hospital because her vision of the left eye sudden dropped 2 months ago. She was examined 2 months ago: visual acuity: 1.0/ 0.5(R/L) IOP: 17.3/ 15(R/L) mmHg. The optic disc of her left eye was pale , visual field showed an inferior fan like defect. Fundus fluorescein angiography(FFA) of her left eye showed ischemic optic neuropathy. the anterior segment, fundus, vision, and FFA of her right eye were normal. She was diagnosed as "left eye ischemic optic neuropathy". She was admitted to our hospital, and examinations showed: visual acuity: 1.0/ 0.15(R/L). IOP: 17.3/ 50.62(R/L), anterior chamber of both eyes were not shallow, Right eye showed no abnormality. Left cornea was mild edema and there was a medium size fat-like KP below the pupil. The boundary of optic papillae in left eye was clear, the color was off white, and the C / D was about 0.3,the angle of left eye was N1 ~ N2. Systemic examination such as X-ray, electrocardiogram and routine laboratory tests were normal. Visual field of right eye was normal and that of the left eye showed a centripetal narrow whit an inferior fan like defect. She was diagnosed as "Left eye PSS,complicated with ischemic optic neuropathy", and treated with drugs for reducing IOP and nutrition curing to optic nerve for about a weak. She was discharged with IOP 12mmHg disappeared KP, vision 0.2 of her left eye. (Clinical data see Figure 22)

Discussion

In 2003 1 case of PSS complicated with nonarteritic anterior ischemic optic neuropathy (AION) was reportd. The vision of the case improved significantly after the attack of PSS had been controlled, but the vision and optic neuropathy damaged continually. The authors emphasized that the IOP of PSS patients complicated with AION should be promptly controlled as it is risk

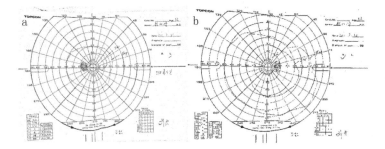

Figure 22. Visual field of patient (Clinical number: 294450) The case suffered from left eye PSS combined with ischemic optic neuropathy. Inferior Visual field defect and serious contraction of left (A),and that of the normal right eye (B).

factors [41]. It is useful to use drugs with dual role of reducing IOP and improving retinal blood supply in intermittent period.

Our case appeared a sudden vision loss and significant discomfort two months ago. The result of examinations in other hospital such as visual field defect of arcuate below and FFA supported the diagnosis of left eye ischemic optic neuropathy. Results of examinations, reaction to treatment and course of the disease during her hospitalization in our hospital In July 2000 conformed with diagnostic criteria of PSS. The structure of the optic nerve , damage of blood vessels and blood state are related to ischemic optic neuropathy, the severely sudden rising of IOP during attack of PSS maybe the inducing factors. So it is necessary to reduce the IOP during each attack of PSS as soon and effective as possible for the cases of PSS combined with ischemic optic neuropathy or with the risk factors for that.

4.3. PSS combined with rhegmatogenous retinal detachment

Typical cases

He was hospitalized in our hospital for the reason that there was shadow before his right eye with a diagnose of rhegmatogenous retinal detachment.

The IOP of his right eye elevated to 29 mmHg 3 days after hospitalization and a fat-like KP appeared in his right eye, than he was diagnosed as rhegmatogenous retinal detachment combined with PSS. Retinal detachment surgery (Condensation + cerclage + scleral pressure technique) were done after reducing IOP with the treatment of drugs.Postoperative recovery was good. PSS recurrenced 4 months later and recovered 5 days late.

Discussion

The pathogenesis of PSS combined with rhegmatogenous retinal detachment is unknown. Increased concentration of PG (especially PGE) resulted from retinal S-antigen entered into the vitreous cavity after blood-eye barrier breakdown during the formation of retinal breaks may leads to the inflammation of the uvea, and the higher concentration of PGs and inflammatory products results in the IOP elevation.

4.4. PSS combined with cataract

Typical cases

She complained of recurrent pain and decreased vision of her right eye for four years.

Results of examinations intraday showed: visual acuity:0.08/ 0.4(R/L); corrected visual acuity R:0.3(-0.75DS/1.50DC*111),L: 0.9(-1.25DS/-0.50DC*83) ;IOP: 12/ 14(R/L) mmHg; a few of timeworn pigmented KP on the central and lower part of her clear corneal; round pupil about 3mm in diameter; normal iris , opacification of posterior capsule of len; C/D of optic papillae o.4.Her left eye appeared normal.

She was hospitalized with the diagnosis of PSS and was treated with carteolol, brimonidine, mannitol for reducing IOP, tobradex for anti-inflammation and methycobal to maintain optic nerve. She was discharged once the attack of PSS faded away every time.The PSS attacked her 1 to 2 month a time, her vision of right eye declined gradually without other discomfort. (Clinical data see Figure 23)

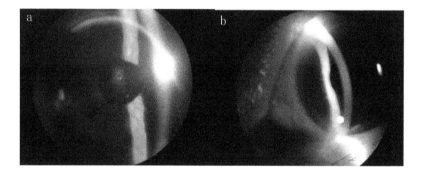

Figure 23. Anterior segment slit-lamp photography of patient (Clinical number: 394998) with the diagnosis of PSS combined with cataract. Arrows show an opacities area at posterior capsule (A) and few typical fat-shaped KPs (B).

5. Discussion

The possible pathogenesis: repeated onset of IOP elevation and anterior segment inflammation cause disorders of nutrition and metabolism of the lens.

Surgical opportunity: Cataract surgery should be done after the inflammation has been subsidized for more than 3 months. The rest of the indication is the same to the conventional cataract.

Author details

He-Zheng Zhou*, Qian Ye, Jian-Guo Wu, Wen-Shan Jiang, Feng Chang, Yan-Ping Song, Qing Ding and Wen-Qiang Zhang

*Address all correspondence to: zhou_h_z@sina.com

Department of Ophthalmology, Wuhan General Hospital, Guangzhou Military Command, Wuhan, China

References

[1] Posener A, Schlossman A. Syndrome of unilateral attacks of glaucoma with cyclic symptoms. Arch opthalmol.1948,39:5-28

[2] Theodore FH. Observation on glaucomatocyclitic crisis(Posner Schloddman Syndrome).Br J Ophthalmol.1952,36:207-213

[3] Dao-Ping Lu, Ran-Ran Xi. [Clinical analyzation of 177 cases with Posner Schloddman Syndrome]. Chin J Ophthalmology. 1982,18:34-37

[4] Paivonsalo HT, Tuminen J, Vaahtoranta LH, et al. Incidence and prevalence of differentuneitis,entilies in Filand. Acta Ophthalmology Scand.1997, 75:76~81.

[5] Kanjiro M. The relationship between elevation of intraocular pressure and prostaglandin in cases with glaucomatocyclitic crisis. clinical ophthalmology. 1975,29:689-692

[6] Yamamoto S, Pavan-Langston D, Tada R, et al. Possible role of herpes simplex virus in the origin of Posner-Schlossman syndrome. Am J Ophthalmol.1995, 119: 796-798

[7] Yang SY, Chen MJ, Chen KH, et al. Cytomegalovirus and herpes simplex virus as causes of bilateral anterior uveitis in an immunocompetent patient. J Chin Med Assoc. 2011,74:48-50

[8] Blich-Michel E, Dussaix E, Cerqueti P, et al. Possible role of cytomegalovirus infection in the etiology of the Posner-Schlossman syndrome. Int Ophthalmol. 1987,11: 95-96

[9] Chee SP, Jap A. Presumed Fuchs heterochromic iridocyclitis and Posner-Schlossman syndrome: comparison of cytomegalovirus-positive and negative eyes. Am 2008,146:883-889

[10] CY Choi, MS Kim, JM Kim, SH Park, KH Park, C Hong. Association between Helicobacter pylori infection and Posner–Schlossman syndrome. Eye. 2010, 24:64-69

[11] Zhi-Hui Li, Xun-Chuan Ji, Shu-Chu Chen, et al. [The Long-term follow-up of Posner Schloddman Syndrome]. Chin J Ophthalmology. 1982,18:306-308

[12] Nan-Xiang Peng. [Clinical analyzation of 52 cases with Posner Schloddman Syndrome].Contemporary Medicine.2008, 5:141-141

[13] Wen-Xue Hu. [Clinical observation of early stage of Posner-Schlossman syndrome]. Int J Ophthalmology. 2011; 11: 1980-1982

[14] Puri P, Verma D. Bilateral glaucomatocyclitic crisis in a patient with Holmes Adie syndrome. J Postgrad Med.1998,44:76-77

[15] Yu-Hong Wang, Xing-Huai Sun. [Clinical analysization of the the the operative effect in patients with glaucomatocyclitic crisis]. Chinese Journal of Practical Ophthalmology. 2005, 10:23-30

[16] Wen-Bing Zhou, Shou-Xiong Peng. [glaucomatocyclitic crisis and Primary Open-angle Glaucoma]. Chinese Ophthalmic Res.1994,12:34-36

[17] He-Zheng Zhou, Yuan-Hong Du. [The related factors about Posner-Schlossman syndrome damage of visual field]. Chinese Journal of Practical Ophthalmology. 2002,10:768~769

[18] Hua-Xin Chen, He-Zheng Zhou, Bai-Chuan Wang et al.[The Clinical Observation of 14 cases elderly Posner-Schlossman syndrome]. Military medical journal of South China. 2007; 21: 43-45

[19] Raitta C, Vannas A. Glaucomatocyclitic crisis. Arch Ophthalmology. 1977, 95:608-612

[20] He-Zheng Zhou, Yi-Jia Yang. [Characteristics and clinical value of the intraocular pressure and the C- value in Posner Schloddman Syndrome]. Chinese Journal of Practical Ophthalmology.1992, 10:143-145

[21] Ying-Bo Shui, Hou-Ren Wei. [Influence of Postural Change on Intraocular Pressure of Normal Eyes]. Chinese Ophthalmic Res. 1987; 3 : 182-185

[22] He-Zheng Zhou. [Tonography and postural change of intraocular pressure in patients with glaucoma]. Chinese Journal of Practical Ophthalmology.1991,9:598-602

[23] He-Zheng Zhou, Wen-Shan Jiang. [Differential diagnosis of Posner-Schlossman syndrome]. Military medical journal of South China.2012,2:32-35

[24] He-Zheng Zhou, Yuan-Hong Du, Yan-Ping Song, Guang-Jie Wang, Jian-Guo Wu. [Visual field damage of glaucomatocyclitic crisis and its relating factors]. Fourth Mil Med Univ.2001,22:1674-1677

[25] Yi-Lin Tang. [Clinical analysis of damage of visual field with Posner Schlossmanps syndrome]. International Journal of Ophthalmology. 2010,10:1204-1205

[26] Jap A, Sivakumar M, Chee SP. Is Posner-Schlossman syndrome benign? Ophthalmology.2001,108:913-991

[27] He-Zheng Zhou, Bai-Chuan Wang, Xiong Zhou. [Unilateral Primary Open-Angle Glaucoma and Bilateral Posner-Schlossman syndrome]. Chin J Misdiagn.2001, 1:334-336

[28] He-Zheng Zhou, Wen-Qiang Zhang, Bai-Chuan Wang. [Glaucomatocyclitic crisis with primary close-Angle glaucoma]. International Journal of Ophthalmology, 2004,4(5):844-847

[29] Darchuk V, Sampaolesi J, Mato L, Nicoli C, Sampaolesi R.Optic nerve head behavior in Posner-Schlossman syndrome. Int Ophthalmol,2001;23:373-379

[30] Rong-Xin Wu. [Operative effect in 1 Case with Posner-Schlossman syndrome].Ocular trauma professional eye disease magazine. 2002,24:328

[31] Lei Sheng, Yu-Pu Li, Gui-Lan Lan. [1 Case of Posner-Schlossman syndrome].Chinese Journal of Practical Ophthalmology.2008,26:572

[32] Bo Zhao, Da-Yong Bai, Hui Zhao.et al. [Posner-Schlossman syndrome and primary open-angle glaucoma]. Chin J Pract Ophthalmology. 2004,22:142-143

[33] Xiu-Feng Ke, Dan-Ning Z, Li Yuan. [Observation the clinical operation curative effect of Posner-Schlossman syndrome]. Chinese Journal of Practical Ophthalmology. 2007,6:642-643

[34] Dinakaran S, Kayarkar V. Trabeculectomy in the management of Posner-Schlossman syndrome. Ophthalmic Surg Lasers.2002,33:321-322

[35] Stavrou P, Murray PI. Does trabeculectomy influence the course of uveitis? Ocul Immunol Inflamm. 1999,7:103-108

[36] Xiao-Ping Zhang, Ji-Zhong Chen, Ru-Yong Song,[Analyze the Diagnostic of Posner-Schlossman syndrome]. Journal of clinical ophthalmology.2002,10:137-139

[37] Jin-Fu Ying, Ling-Ling Wu, [Posner-Schlossman syndrome complicated with Primary Closed-Angle Glaucoma]. Chinese Journal of Practical Ophthalmology. 1993.11:491-492

[38] Chang-lin Zhao, Han-Ping Xie. [A case report of primary angle closure glaucoma accompanied by glaucomatocyclitic crisis]. Acta Academiae Medicinae Militaris Tertiae. 2004.10.25; 26: 1798

[39] Li-Hong Guan. [2 cases of Posner-Schlossman syndrome complicated with Primary Closed-Angle Glaucoma]. Modern Medicine & Health. 2008,24:152

[40] Wen-Shan Jiang, He-Zheng Zhou,Yun-Hui Chen, Ling Hong [Differential diagnosis of the Posner-Schlossman syndrome with heterochromic iris and the Fuchs syndrome—clinial report about three cases].International Journal of Ophthalmology, 2009;9(9):1762-1763

[41] Irak I, Katz BJ, Zabriskie NA, Zimmerman PL.Posner-Schlossman syndrome and nonarteritic anterior ischemic optic neuropathy. J Neuroophthalmol. 2003,23: 264-267

Progressive Neurodegeneration of Retina in Alzheimer's Disease — Are β-Amyloid Peptide and Tau New Pathological Factors in Glaucoma?

Kin Chiu, Kwok-Fai So and
Raymond Chuen-Chung Chang

Additional information is available at the end of the chapter

1. Introduction

Alzheimer's disease (AD) is a neurodegenerative disease affecting 5.4 million people globally and is predicated to affect over 100 million people worldwide by 2050 [1]. It is the most common form of progressive cognitive decline. As originally described by Alois Alzheimer in 1907, AD is associated with extracellular amyloid plaque formation and intracellular neurofibrillary tangles in the brain regions involved in learning and memory processes [2]. A major problem of the disease is, perhaps, altered proteolytic processing of the amyloid precursor protein (APP) resulting in the production and aggregation of neurotoxic forms of Aβ. Amyloid plaques are extracellular deposits of fibrils and amorphous aggregates of β-amyloid (Aβ). Compact plaques have been considered to be associated with neuronal and synaptic loss, dystrophic neurites, hypertrophic astrocytes, activated microglia cells, and various features of inflammatory processes. The intracellular neurofibrillary tangles consist of paired helical filaments formed by the microtubule-associated protein tau that exhibits hyperphosphorylation and oxidative modifications. Increasing lines of evidence have shown that visual impairment is associated with the prevalence of AD [3]-[5].

Glaucoma is recognized as an age-related neurodegenerative disorder – optic neuropathy. Being the second leading cause of blindness, it is estimated that glaucoma will affect more than 80 million people worldwide with at least 6 - 8 million individuals becoming bilaterally blind by the year 2020 [6]. Comparing to normal population, the prevalence of glaucoma is about 2.5 times higher in AD patients [7]. In 2011, Nucci and co-workers reported that glaucoma progression was associated with altered levels of Aβ and tau proteins in cerebral spinal fluid

[8]. The intravitreous levels of $A\beta_{1-42}$ are significantly decreased and that of tau are markedly increased in glaucoma patients [9]. We propose that accumulation of $A\beta$ and hyperphosphorylated tau protein should be considered to be new pathological factors to propagate neurodegeneration in glaucoma.

1.1. Amyloid precursor protein and functions

APP is a type I transmembrane protein with a single transmembrane domain, a large extracellular ectodomain, and a short cytoplasmic tail [10]. The processing of APP to $A\beta$ is an important event in the pathogenesis of AD [11]. The processing is initiated by cleavage of APP by α-secretase within the $A\beta$ region, and by cleavage by β-secretase (BACE) at the amino terminus of $A\beta$, leading to the secretion of large soluble ectodomains. In pathological situation, if the carboxyl-terminal fragments is processed by γ-secretase resulting in the production of $A\beta$, p3, and the APP intracellular domain (AICD). In humans, the *APP* gene is located on chromosome 21 with three major isoforms (APP695, APP751 and APP770) arising from alternative splicing [12]. APP is highly expressed in neurons where the protein is rapidly transported down the axons to nerve terminus in the brain and retina [13].

As the processing of APP to $A\beta$ is an important event in the pathogenesis of AD, great effort has been devoted to understand biological functions of APP since its cloning in 1988 [10]. In vitro and in vivo studies have shown important activities of APP in modulating neurite outgrowth [14], synaptic activity [15]-[17], metal homeostasis [18], [19], synaptic transmission [20] and synaptic adhesion at the neuromuscular junction [21]. In retina, APP plays a role in retinogenesis. In APP knockout (KO) mice, differentiation of some inner retinal neurons, specifically horizontal and amacrine cells are hampered in APP-KO mice during early postnatal development[22]. However, normal numbers of horizontal cells and most types of amacrine cells are found in adult APP-KO mice. The number is similar to adult C57/B6JxSV129 wild type control mice. APP is expressed in inner retina including horizontal, cone bipolar, amacrine and ganglion cells in the APP-KO mice. Although APP is not required for gross retinal structure or visual acuity in adult retina, it is required for the inner retinal function of the rod and cone pathway [23].

1.2. Tau protein and functions

1.2.1. Tau protein

Tau protein is microtubule-associated protein that stabilizes microtubules and able to form aggregation in pathological conditions. Tau is expressed from the gene known as microtubule-associated protein tau (MAPT) on chromosome 17 at position 17q21. Tau is highly expressed in neurons and is abundant in axons [24]. Hyperphosphorylated, insoluble, and filamentous tau proteins were shown to be the main component of neurofibrillary tangles (NFTs), a pathological hallmark of AD [24].

Tau binding to microtubules enables them to play a fundamental role in promoting microtubule assembly and stability; and in turn, affecting intra-neuronal transport of cargos. Detachment of tau from microtubules leads to dysfunction of axonal transport and even retraction of spines[25]. Apart from stabilizing microtubules, tau has a more versatile role in the central nervous system (CNS). Tau regulates the process of neurite extension via its ability to stop microtubule-severing proteins and its facilitative role on nerve growth factor signaling [26]. Tau interacts via its amino-terminal projection domain with the kinase Fyn (a proto-oncogene tyrosine-protein kinase). Fyn phosphorylates the N-methyl-D-aspartate receptor (NMDAR) to link NMDAR to synaptic excitotoxic downstream signaling [27]. Recent findings also reported that Tau can modulate phospholipase C gamma [28], histone deacetylase-6 [29], and heat shock proteins [30]. Tau also interacts with actin via acidic N-terminals, projecting from microtubules for neurite outgrowth and stabilization during the brain development [31]. In tau knockout mice, neurogenesis is severely reduced [32].

1.2.2. Multiple functions of tau in the retina

In the retina, tau not only regulates the cytoskeleton and axonal transport in retinal neurons, but also affects accumulation of Aβ and cell survival signaling. The pivotal roles of tau in retinal functions are summarized in Figure 1.

It has been found that tau is expressed in a gradient manner in retinal ganglion cells (RGC), with higher levels in the terminal parts of axons of developing RGCs. Its localization at the axon plays a role in proper axon development and survival of RGCs [33]. Exposure to okadaic acid resulted in accumulation of phosphorylated tau, followed by distortion of the cytoskeleton leading to growth cone collapse. Hence, tau has been implicated in the process of establishing neuronal axon polarity [34]. Interruption in these transport mechanisms would cause the accumulation of Aβ, which can propagate secondary degeneration. Studies based on Tg2576 transgenic mice showed that immunoreactivity of hyperphosphorylated tau was found to be very close to that of Aβ in mouse retina [35].

Tau can be phosphorylated by cyclin-dependent kinase 5 (Cdk5), a proline-directed serine/ threonine kinase. Phosphorylation leads tau to dissociate from microtubules and affects its stability. Cdk5 is highly expressed in neuronal axons and growth cones serving to promote neurite outgrowth and migration[36]. To initiate its activation, Cdk5 requires interaction with its activator subunit p35. Cdk5 has been implicated to phosphorylate various substrates to regulate a diverse range of cellular processes in the CNS. Studies have shown that ephrin-A signaling pathway can also lead to the activation of Cdk5. Ephrin-A regulates retinotectal projection via receptor-mediated axon growth repulsion through a complex signaling cascade. Fyn can activate Cdk5 to phosphorylate collapsin response mediator protein (CRMP2) to reduce microtubule assembly[37]. Immunofluorescence studies have shown that activation of Cdk5 occurs downstream of ephrin-A5 signaling to phosphorylate tau in the growth cones and axons of RGCs. These findings suggest that phosphorylation of tau serves as another means to which ephrin-A signaling can induce microtubule reorganization in RGC growth cones[38].

Apart from Cdk5, tau has also been found to interact with calcium/calmodulin-dependent protein kinase II (CaMKII) in the CaMKII-α-associated protein complex in chick retina. Endogenous association of tau with CaMKII-α suggests that it is important in regulating

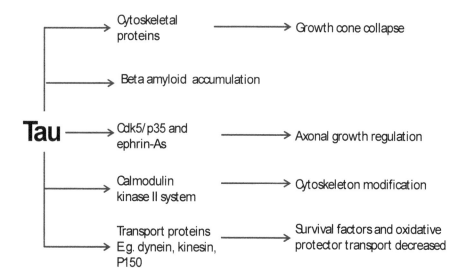

Figure 1. Schematic diagram summarizing the roles of tau in retinal functions. Tau stabilizes microtubules. Dislocation of Tau from microtubules can result in growth cone collapse. Accumulation of β-amyloid (Aβ) is an example to trigger phosphorylation of tau and hence detaches from microtubule. Apart from Aβ as a triggering factor, any stimulation of signaling cascade of cdk5, ephrin-A receptor or calmodulin-dependent protein kinase II affecting phosphorylation of tau can also modulate microtubules. Once tau leaves microtubules after phosphorylation, they can easily form aggregation, which can further impair axonal transport mediated by kinesin or dynein. Consequently, mitochondria in the distal part of nerve, nerve terminus or spines cannot obtain protection from the cell body (soma) so that they are collapse and cannot produce energy. Neurodegeneration can unavoidably occur.

cytoskeletal assembly in neurons. Through the phosphorylation of tau, microtubule assembly may be inhibited; and hence, the cellular architecture is disrupted[39].

Abnormally aggregated tau inhibits the transportation of mitochondria by kinesin-like motors towards the cell periphery of rat RGCs. Consequently, neurons with perturbation of mitochondria and peroxisomes suffer from loss of energy production and accumulation of reactive oxygen species (ROS). The anterograde transport of vesicles required for growth cones and synaptic function is retarded. In addition, these neurons may be more vulnerable to oxidative stress[40]. In the RGCs axons of P301S mutant mice, the projection domain of tau interacts with the C-terminus of p150, the major component of the dynein-activator. The co-localization of tau and p150 suggests that tau dysfunction can result in the mislocalization of dynactin in axons, which can result in neurodegeneration[41].

2. Clinical manifestation of visual deficits in Alzheimer's patients

Various visual deficits in AD have been reported since 1987 [42]. Cognitive visual changes have been reported in patients in the early stages of AD [43], including difficulties in reading and finding objects [44]-[46], depth perception [43] perceiving structure from motion [44], [46]-[48], color recognition [44], [49], and impairment in spatial contrast sensitivity [47], [50]. Previously, these changes have been attributed to neuronal damage to the visual pathways in the brain rather than the retina [51]. However, there are increasing lines of evidence showing that specific AD like pathology (amyloid plaques and NFT) in the brain can be found in the retina. In 2011, Koronyn-Hamaoui and co-workers [52] identified amyloid plaques in the retinas from AD patients as well as patients in mild cognitive impairment.

Cross-sectional imaging of the retina using optical coherence tomography (OCT) has demonstrated a significant reduction of thickness in peripapillary retinal fiber layer (RFL) of patients with early AD when compared with age-matched controls[53]-[57]. The thinning of RFL was observed predominantly in the inferior and superior quadrants, which was consistent with the inferior and superior visual field loss in AD patients[44], [54]. Reduction of the macular thickness has also been reported in AD; and the total volume of the macula is inversely correlated with the severity of the disease[55]. Changes in the optic nerve head have been observed using confocal scanning laser ophthalmoscopy (cSLO). The observed changes include reduced RFL thickness, neuroretinal rim volume and area, and increased cup-disc ratio; suggesting an overall reduction in the number of optic nerve fibers passing through the optic nerve head [58]. These *in vivo* findings are corroborated by the histopathological findings of axonal degeneration in optic nerves, reduced thickness of RFL and a significant reduction in the number of large diameter RGCs in the post-mortem AD retinas [59], [60].

According to the definitions of glaucoma published in 2002 by an international consensus panel [61], glaucoma is thought to be present when at least one eye has typical defects both in structural and functional aspects (optic disc damage and visual field loss, respectively) [62]. Characteristically, the damage indicates the death of RGC in the inner retina and loss of axons in the optic nerve. This structural loss of the axons can be recognized clinically by ophthalmoscope or can be detected by imaging devices such as OCT and scanning laser polarimetry. Besides NFL thinning, the similarities between the ocular effects of AD and glaucoma can be observed in pattern electroretinogram (PERG) responses [63], [64], the type of cell loss (large magnocellular RGC) and possibly the mechanisms for loss of RGC (apoptosis) [65], [66]. This may explain the high incidence of glaucoma in AD patients [7], [67]. The involvement of Aβ accumulation and hyperphosphorylated tau protein might be important causes of neurodegneration of RGCs in glaucoma.

3. Retinal degeneration in AD transgenic mice

Since there is a lack of postmortem human retinal samples from AD patients, progress of investigating pathogenesis of retinal neurodegeneration in the AD eyes is slow. Much of the insights have gained from specific gene mutations that account for the familial AD (FAD). The majority (30-40%) of FAD is resulted from autosomal dominant inheritance with mutated genes encoding presenilin 1 (PS1) on the long arm of chromosome 14, presenilin 2 (PS2) on chromosome 1 and amyloid precursor protein (APP) on chromosome 21 [68].

Depending on the number of genes they express, transgenic mice come in three varieties: single (APP, PS1, or Tau), double (APP/PS1, APP/Tau), or triple transgenic (APP/PS1/ Tau) [69]. Behavioral studies on AD transgenic mice showed that the mice were suffered from visual dysfunction [70].

Multiple lines of AD transgenic mice have elicited AD-like pathological hallmarks in the retina as disease progresses [69]. The over-expression of APP, the production of soluble Aβ, and Aβ deposition will lead to formation of amyloid plaques that can induce cell death via the apoptotic pathway [71]. Even before formation of plaques, oligomeric Aβ can induce synaptic degeneration. Furthermore, Aβ plays a role in inducing hyperphosphorylation of tau, which in turn affects the integrity of retinal cells and their synapses in inner nuclear layer (INL) [72]. It has been reported that over-expression of APP, Aβ and/or tau deposition, neuronal cell loss, changes of retinal glial cell, and vascular changes occur in the retina of AD transgenic mice. The changes of retinal histopathology documented in the AD transgenic mouse models are summarized in Table 1.

3.1. Loss of retinal neurons in AD transgenic mice

In consistent with the findings in the retina of AD patient, reduced retinal thickness between RGCL and ONL was detected in Tg2576 mice [73]. This indicates that there was a loss of either the photoreceptor cells in the ONL (rod and cone cells) or neuronal cells in the inner retinal layers (RGC, horizontal cells, bipolar cells or amacrine cells). In double transgenic mice strain (APP$_{swe}$/PS1$_{M146L}$), a significant increase in the number of apoptotic cells in the RGCL was detected by TUNEL staining as the animal grew from 7.8 months to 27 months [11]. By using a different double transgenic mice strain (APPswe/PS1$_{\Delta E9}$), there was significant increase of TUNEL-positive cells in the RGCL when comparing with age-matched controls. Most recently, direct visualization of apoptotic RGCs in the retina was reported in triple transgenic mouse model of AD [74]. Using a fluorophore-labeled annexin V protein as a marker of apoptosis and cSLO to detect the fluorescence, the triple transgenic mice displayed increased number of RGC apoptosis compared with wild-type controls.

3.2. Over-expression of APP in the AD retina

Compared to the wild-type mice, a significant increase in immunoreactivity of APP in the cytoplasm was detected in RGCL and INL of various transgenic mice [11], [73], [74]. In single transgenic Tg2576 mice, over expressed APP was detected in the RGCL and INL of 14-month-old mice [73], [75]. In double transgenic mice strain APP$_{swe}$/PS1$_{M146L}$, over-expression of APP was age-dependent. In 27 months old mice, immunoreactivity of APP was detected not only in the different layers of retina such as NFL, RGCL, inner plexiform layer (IPL), INL, outer plexiform layer (OPL), outer segment (OS) and retinal pigment epithelium (RPE) but also in the retinal vasculature [11]. By using different double transgenic strain- APP$_{swe}$/PS1$_{\Delta E9}$, APP immunoreactivity was exhibited in the RGCL only at an intermediate age of 10.5 months. In earlier time point (9 month-old animals), moderate immunoreactivity of APP was detected only in the IPL and OPL not in the RGCL [11], [73], [76], [77].

3.3. Deposition of Aβ in the retina and retinal vasculature

The deposition of Aß, derived from abnormal processing of APP was found in the retinas of AD transgenic mice. In single transgenic Tg2576 mice, Aβ was found to deposit from RGCL to INL or even at ONL. Aβ deposits and plaque like formation were detected by four different monoclonal antibodies such as BAM01, 6E10, Aβ-40 and Aβ-42 as well as Congo red staining[73], [76]. Retinal Aβ deposit has also been found in double transgenic mouse models expressing APP/PS1.

Mutant genes	Type/ Age	Neuronal cell loss^	APP over-expression	Aβ deposits	Aβ-deposited vasculature	P-tau deposits	Ref.
APP$_{swe}$ (HuAPP695. K670N, M671L)	Single/ 14-months	Yes	+++ (GCL, INL)	+++ (GCL, IPL, INL, OPL, ONL, RV) + (OS)	Yes	± (GCL, IPL, INL, OPL, ONL)	[73]
APP$_{swe}$ (HuAPP695. K595N, M596L)	Single/ 2-to18-months	n/a	+++ (GCL, INL)	± (GCL, RV)	Yes	n/a	[75]
APP$_{swe}$, PS1$_{ΔE9}$	Double/ 6-to 12-months	n/a	++ (IPL, OPL)	± (GCL, INL, RV)	Yes	n/a	[75]
APP$_{swe}$, PS1$_{ΔE9}$	Double/ 10.5-months	Yes	+++ (GCL)	± (NFL,CV)	Yes	n/a	[11]
APP$_{swe}$, PS1$_{ΔE9}$	Double/ 12-to 19-months	No	n/a	*(IPL, OPL)	n/a	n/a	[77]
APP$_{swe}$, PS1$_{M146L}$	Double/ 7.8 months	Yes	+ (GCL, INL)		Yes	n/a	[11]
APP$_{swe}$, PS1$_{M146L}$	Double/ 27-months	Yes	+++ (NFL,GCL, IPL, INL, OPL, + OS, RPE, RV)	+++ (NFL, GCL) (RV, CV)	Yes	n/a	[11]
TauP301S	Single/ 1- to 6-months	No	n/a	n/a	n/a	±(IPL), with paired helical filament formation	[78]
PS1$_{M146V}$, APP$_{swe}$, and TauP301L	Triple/ 10-to 22-months	Yes	n/a	*Yes (layers not specified)	n/a	n/a	[79]

n/a: not applicable; *swe*: Swedish mutation; *P-tau*: hyperphosphorylated tau; ^ neuronal cells in the inner retinal regions, including INL and GCL; * plaques formation; *NFL*: nerve fiber layer; *GCL*: ganglion cell layer; *IPL*: inner plexiform layer; *INL*: inner nuclear layer; *OPL*: outer plexiform layer; *ONL*: outer nuclear layer; *OS*: outer segment; *RPE*: retinal pigment epithelium; *RV*: retinal vasculature; *CV*: choroidal vasculature; +++ strong level; ++ moderate level; + weak level; +/- present.

Table 1. Retinal changes in documented AD transgenic mouse models

In double transgenic mice strain $APP_{swe}/PS1_{M146L}$, Aβ was found to deposit predominantly in NFL and RGCL in aged mice of 27 months but not at young mice of 7.8 months. In another double transgenic strain $APP_{swe}/PS1_{\Delta E9}$, similar A$\beta$ deposition was detected in intermediate age of 10.5 months[11]. In another subsequent study using transgenic mice APPswe/PS1ΔE9, Aβ plaques were found by thioflavin-S staining in plexiform layers; the size and the number of plaques significantly increased with age from 12 months[77]. The transparent nature of the eyes allows direct tracking and visualization of the Aβ signal has also been detected in the retinal and choroidal vasculature. In single transgenic Tg2576 mice, Aβ was detected around microvessels in RGCL[73], [76]. Both retinal and choroidal vascular Aβ deposits were reported in aged (27 months) $APP_{swe}/PS1_{M146L}$ transgenic mice and intermediate-aged (10.5 months) $APP_{swe}/PS1_{\Delta E9}$ mice [11].

3.4. Deposition of hyperphosphorylated tau in the retina

Hyperphosphorylation of tau protein and subsequent deposition as neurofilbrillary tangles is associated with AD. Tau inclusions have been observed in the brains as well as in the retinas of Tg2576 and triple transgenic mice [79]. In single transgenic Tg2576 mice, hyperphosphory-lated tau was detected by antibody AT8 in various retinal layers from RGCL through to the ONL. The hyperphosphorylated tau was found to be associated with Aβ depositions [73]. Another single transgenic expresses human P301S tau transgene, hyperphosphorylated tau was found to deposit in the RNFL and aggregated into filamentous inclusions in RGCs starting from 2-month-old mice [78]. Hyperphosphorylation and aggregation of tau were associated *in vivo* with reduced axonal transport, both anterograde and retrograde, in the optic nerve of this transgenic mice line [80].

3.5. Glial reaction in AD retina

Glial reactions, activated microglia and astrocytes, in the retina were detected in different kinds of AD transgenic mice at various ages. In Tg2576 transgenic mice, significant infiltration of microglial cells detected by iba-1 and the increased astrocytes activation detected by GFAP in the inner retina were detected as early as 4-month-old mice [73]. In double transgenic $APP_{swe}/PS1_{M146L}$ mice, microglia was increased in an age-dependent manner, which was in parallel with Aβ deposits and TUNEL positive RGC in the GCL. The average percentage of cells in the GCL surrounded by microglial cells increased significantly from 10% in 7.8-month-old to 50% in 27-month-old $APP_{swe}/PS1_{M146L}$ transgenic mice [11]. In another double transgenic $APP_{swe}/PS1_{\Delta E9}$ mice, qualitative evaluation revealed greater immunoreactivity of microglia in 12 to 19 months old transgenic mice when compared to age-matched non-transgenic control[77].

4. β-Amyloid peptide and glaucoma

4.1. Aβ in animal models mimic glaucoma

In a rat model mimicking chronic ocular hypertension (COH) [81], Aβ has been reported to be implicated in the development of RGC apoptosis in glaucoma. Increased intracellular Aβ in

RGC detected by using Aβ antibody was co-localized with apoptotic RGC cells. Targeting Aβ pathway in this experimental model, three different approaches were applied including: (i) β-secretase inhibitor to reduce formation of Aβ; (ii) an anti-Aβ antibody to clear Aβ deposition; and (iii) Congo red to inhibit aggregation of Aβ and neurotoxic effects of Aß. Manipulating production of Aβ pathway, apoptosis of RGC was successfully reduced by suppressing further Aβ aggregation and inhibiting the enzymatic activity of amyloidogenesis. The combined treatment (triple therapy) was more effective than either single- or dual-agent therapy in protecting RGC survival under COH. Increased expression of Aβ in the RGCL and optic nerve was related to abnormal APP-splicing in the presence of elevated IOP in DBA/2J glaucomatous mouse retinas [82] and mouse experimental COH model [83]. Increase of Aβ in the retinal in COH has been found to be associated with activation of caspase-8 and caspase-3, and caspase-3-mediated APP cleavage product (DeltaC-APP) in the RGCs under COH [65]. Application of exogenous Aβ peptide into the vitreous also induced significant RGC apoptosis in rat retina [81].

4.2. Aβ-mediated mitochondrial dysfunction and glaucoma

There are some suggestions that Aβ peptides modulate Ca^{2+} level in mitochondria that may alter the mitochondrial morphology and physiology [84]. For examples, elevated cytosolic Ca^{2+} levels may enhance fragmentation of mitochondria. This can lead to the perturbation of fission and fusion balance, which may eventually cause mitochondrial dysfunction [85]. Dysregulation of Ca^{2+} homeostasis may also disrupt downstream pathways of Ca^{2+}-dependent regulators monitoring mitochondrial dynamics [84], [86]. Consequently, synaptic dysfunction may occur due to the failure of meeting the energy demand in neurons, particularly in axonal and dendritic terminals [86]-[88].

Our eyes are energy demanding organs in which high density of mitochondria exist at the optic nerve heads [89]. If one applies Aβ to the eyes, it may trigger mitochondrial dysfunctions resulting in retinal degeneration. Intriguingly, in a glaucomatous model where cultured RGCs were subjected to elevated hydrostatic pressure, fission of mitochondria was found to be enhanced, together with morphological changes and bioenergetics dysfunction [90]. A clinical study showed that mean mitochondrial respiratory activity was decreased by 21% in patients with primary open-angle glaucoma compared with age-matched control subjects (p < 0.001) [91]. In rabbit model of COH, daily tropical application of 5 µM mitochondria targeted cationic plastoquinone derivative SkQ1 (10-(6'-plastoquinonyl) decyltriphenylphosphonium) showed reduction in glaucomatous changes [92]. This hypothesis may be extended to one of the causes in Aβ-induced RGC apoptosis in glaucoma.

5. TAU and glaucoma

5.1. Tau in the retina of glaucoma patient

In aged retina (49-87 year-old human), there is a positive correlation between age and number of tau-positive RGCs. Diffuse immunoreactivity of tau was found in the INL, while aggregated tau was found within the cytoplasm of photoreceptor cells in patients older than 63-years-old [93]. Total tau is present in the INL and IPL but much reduced in glaucomatous retina. On the other hand, phosphorylated Tau (pTau) recognized by monoclonal antibody-AT8 is detected in glaucomatous retina at the outer border of the INL and occasionally in the IPL. It has also been found that pTau was localized in horizontal cells labeled by cell marker-parvalbumin [94]. The distribution of tau in the normal aged (Fig. 2A) and glaucomatous retina (Fig. 2B) is summarized in Figure 2. The decrease of total Tau and accumulation of pTau in the glaucomatous retina support the hypothesis showing that glaucoma shares pathways with AD. This is consistent with previous reports showing an increased incidence of primary open-angle glaucoma among AD patients. Recent evidence also indicates that altered cerebrospinal fluid (CSF) circulatory dynamics can reduce the clearance of both Aβ and tau. Altered CSF circulatory dynamics can reduce clearance of neurotoxin along the optic nerve in the subarachnoid space; leading to deposition of tau and other toxic molecules which ultimately result in glaucoma progression[94].

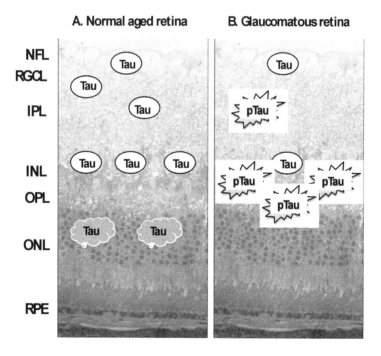

Figure 2. Diagram summarizing the literature reporting on the distribution of tau in the retina of normal people (A) and glaucomatous patient (B). The background is a cross semi-thin section showing the layered structure of the retina. *Ovals labelled 'Tau'* represent expression of total tau. *Cloudy labelled 'Tau'* represent tau aggregates. *Sparckle labelled 'pTau'* represent expression of abnormal phosphorylated tau. NFL: nerve fiber layer, RGCL: retinal ganglion cell layer, IPL: inner plexiform layer, INL: inner nuclear layer, OPL: outer plexiform layer, ONL: outer nuclear layer, RPE: retinal pigment epithelium.

5.2. Tau in animal models mimic glaucoma

In human glaucoma (chronic ocular hypertension), decreased total Tau and increased phosphorylated tau (pTau) are reported when compared to the age control group [94]. In animal models mimicking acute ocular hypertension, the loss of tau is evident even at earlier stages when the outer layer of the retina is mostly intact [95]. Acute ocular hypertension was induced for 1 hour by elevation of IOP to 120 mm Hg. The loss of tau proteins in the retina has been shown to occur from as early as 4 hours to over 7 days after induction of acute ocular hypertension. Proteolysis of tau has been suggested contributing to the pathogenesis of neuronal cell death, correlating with an increase in calcium, followed by activation of calpain. Calpain-induced conversion of p35 to p25 and activation of cdk5 are also involved in the RGC loss. There is no direct evidence about increase of pTau. However, it is indirectly evident by the up-regulation of the relevant kinase, cdk5, and the regulatory protein, p35/p25. One justification for the failure to detect pTau is that tau protein is cleaved by calpain before detection is possible [95]. Another justification is that this acute elevation of ocular hypertension actually blocks the retinal blood supply at 120 mmHg IOP. This is an ischemia/reperfusion model which may cause neuronal cell hypoxia. Under hypoxic conditions, similar changes have also been reported. In rat retinas treated with hypoxic conditions, it has been found that immunoreactivity of tau is almost completely lost in retinas within 5 hours; however, the proteolytic products of tau remain detectable [96]. The changes of Tau proteins in the chronic ocular hypertension model which mimic glaucoma over a relative long and slow degenerative period deserves further evaluation.

6. Future therapy

Increasing lines of evidence have demonstrated common pathological findings in both AD and glaucomatous retinal degeneration. Neuronal losses, inflammatory responses, accumulation of Aβ and pTau deposition are important pathological factors found in the brain and the retina [94], [97]. However, the correlation among Aβ deposits, pTau formation and the retinal degeneration is limited to histological level. The pathological mechanisms have not been comprehensively investigated. Questions like what are the mechanisms triggered by Aβ and tau to cause retinal degeneration are still waiting for answers.

As part of the CNS, the similarity between the brain and the retina allows the exchange of knowledge in terms of pathological mechanisms and therapeutic intervention. Mitochondrial dysfunction discussed above is one of the pathophysiological changes in both AD and retinal degeneration [3], [98]. The discovery of significant involvement of double-stranded RNA-dependent protein kinase (PKR) in the apoptosis of neurons in postmortem AD brain and in experimental studies is another good example [99]-[101]. Years after our report of the PKR in AD, PKR has also been proved to play important roles in neuronal apoptosis of RGCs in endoplasmic reticulum (ER) stress-induced retinal neuronal loss [102]. Neuroprotective agents found from *in vitro* AD research can also be applied to eye research. Our Studies on wolfberry, *Lycium barbarum*, an anti-aging herb, can be a good example. In primary neuronal culture, wolfberry can alleviate the Aβinduced degenerative process by promoting survival signals, suppressing ER stress, reducing glutamate excitotoxicity [103]-[107]. In rat glaucoma model, wolfberry shows its beneficial effects on the retina based on suppressing neurodestructive factors, modulating the inflammatory responses [108], and up regulating the expression of protective chaperone – crystallin [109]. The neuroprotective effects of wolfberry shared between AD and glaucoma further strengthen our hypothesis that knowledge obtained from the brain can be transferred to the study of the retina.

On the other hand, retina can be a promising platform to investigate the efficacy of any potential drugs on different neuronal cells. In the study of rat chronic glaucomatous model, immunotherapy with a potential agent such as β-secretase inhibitor, Congo Red or Aβ antibody successfully reduced Aβ-induced RGC apoptosis by suppressing further Aβ aggregation and inhibiting the enzymatic activity of amyloidogenesis [81]. In APPswe/PS1ΔE9 mice, following MOG45D-loaded dendritic cells immunization, Aβ–plaque burden in the retinas was reduced as effective as that in the brain [52].

In a recent study using APPswe/PS1ΔE9 mice with five days of systemic administration of curcumin, the results showed that there is a age-dependent correlation between plaque deposition in the retina and the brain, and increased accumulations over the course of disease progression [52]. This is the very first prove that Aβ plaques in the retina pre-cede the existence of brain plaques. The Aβ plaques can be detected as early as 2.5 months of age in the retina but Aβ plaques in the brain exists at the age of 5 months, which is about 2 months later [110]. Curcumin is a natural and safe fluorochrome that binds and labels Aβ plaques [111], [112]. In a six-month randomized, placebo-controlled, double-blind, pilot clinical trial in AD patients, there was no significant side effects even when patients took curcumin at the dose of 4 g/day [113].

Early sign of AD symptoms in the brain can hardly be detected. With the use of curcumin, retinal degeneration may be the most important site to be studied in early AD pathology. Future development of high-resolution optical imaging for early AD diagnosis, prognosis assessment and response to therapies can be achieved non-invasively through direct imaging of the retina. Progression of therapy is possible to be visualized qualitatively in a sense that one can monitor the changes of a particular neuronal cell [114], [115]. Quantitative examination of the disease stages have been performed by assessing the ratio of apoptosis to necrosis using fluorescence counts of respective dyes [74]. Even more, a high spatial resolution of images with a high signal-to-noise ratio ranging from 3:1 to 10:1 can be achieved with the imaging of the retina [114], [115]. The merits of non-invasive retinal imaging can provide investigators a solid support for assessing pathological status as well as developing and refining therapeutic strategies. Considering the potential of direct optical imaging of the retina, especially the Aβ plaques deposition in the retina labeled by curcumin, retinal degeneration in early AD is the window of monitoring disease progression as well as effectiveness of treatment.

With all the findings we pointed out in this review, we can formulate our working hypothesis for researchers: increase in the level of Aβ or hyperphosphorylated tau protein may be the co-pathological factors of glaucoma leading to progressive neurodegeneration in the retina.

Acknowledgements

Research in this laboratory is partly supported by HKU Alzheimer's Disease Research Network under Strategic Research Theme on Healthy Aging. The authors declare that we do not have competing interest in this review.

Author details

Kin Chiu[1], Kwok-Fai So[1,2,3] and Raymond Chuen-Chung Chang[1,2,3]

1 Laboratory of Neurodegenerative Diseases, Department of Anatomy, LKS Faculty of Medicine, China

2 Research Centre of Heart, Brain, Hormone and Healthy Aging, LKS Faculty of Medicine, China

3 State Key Laboratory of Brain and Cognitive Sciences, The University of Hong Kong, Pokfulam, Hong Kong SAR, China

References

[1] Brookmeyer R, Johnson E, Ziegler-Graham K, HM A. Forecasting the global burden of Alzheimer's disease. Alzheimers Dement 2007;3:186-191.

[2] Mattson MP. Pathways towards and away from Alzheimer's disease. Nature 2004;430:631-639.

[3] Valenti DA. Alzheimer's disease: visual system review. Optometry 2010;81:12-21.

[4] Berisha F, Feke GT, Trempe CL, McMeel JW, Schepens CL. Retinal abnormalities in early Alzheimer's disease. Invest Ophthalmol Vis Sci 2007;48:2285-2289.

[5] Rizzo M, Anderson SW, Dawson J, Nawrot M. Vision and cognition in Alzheimer's disease. Neuropsychologia 2000;38:1157-1169.

[6] Quigley HA, Broman AT. The number of people with glaucoma worldwide in 2010 and 2020. British J Ophthalmol 2006;90:262-267.

[7] Tamura H, Kawakami H, Kanamoto T, et al. High frequency of open-angle glaucoma in Japanese patients with Alzheimer's disease. J Neurol Sci 2006;246:79-83.

[8] Nucci C, Martucci A, Martorana A, Sancesario GM, Cerulli L. Glaucoma progression associated with altered cerebral spinal fluid levels of amyloid beta and tau proteins. Clin Exp Ophthalmol 2011;39:279-281.

[9]   Yoneda S, Hara H, Hirata A, Fukushima M, Inomata Y, Tanihara H. Vitreous fluid
      levels of beta-amyloid((1-42)) and tau in patients with retinal diseases. Jpn J Ophthal-
      mol 2005;49:106-108.

[10] Muller UC, Zheng H. Physiological Functions of APP Family Proteins. Cold Spring
      Harb Perspect Med 2012;2:a006288.

[11] Ning A, Cui J, To E, Ashe KH, Matsubara J. Amyloid-beta deposits lead to retinal de-
      generation in a mouse model of Alzheimer disease. Invest Ophthalmol Vis Sci
      2008;49:5136-5143.

[12] Goate A, Chartier-Harlin MC, Mullan M, et al. Segregation of a missense mutation in
      the amyloid precursor protein gene with familial Alzheimer's disease. Nature
      1991;349:704-706.

[13] Chow VW, Mattson MP, Wong PC, Gleichmann M. An overview of APP processing
      enzymes and products. Neuromolecular Med 2010;12:1-12.

[14] Hoe H-S, Lee KJ, Carney RSE, et al. Interaction of Reelin with Amyloid Precursor
      Protein Promotes Neurite Outgrowth. J Neurosci 2009;29:7459-7473.

[15] Priller C, Bauer T, Mitteregger G, Krebs B, Kretzschmar HA, Herms J. Synapse for-
      mation and function is modulated by the amyloid precursor protein. J Neurosci
      2006;26:7212-7221.

[16] Moya KL, Benowitz LI, Schneider GE, Allinquant B. The amyloid precursor protein
      is developmentally regulated and correlated with synaptogenesis. Dev Biol
      1994;161:597-603.

[17] Herard AS, Besret L, Dubois A, et al. siRNA targeted against amyloid precursor pro-
      tein impairs synaptic activity in vivo. Neurobiol Aging 2006;27:1740-1750.

[18] White AR, Reyes R, Mercer JF, et al. Copper levels are increased in the cerebral cortex
      and liver of APP and APLP2 knockout mice. Brain Res 1999;842:439-444.

[19] Duce JA, Tsatsanis A, Cater MA, et al. Iron-export ferroxidase activity of beta-amy-
      loid precursor protein is inhibited by zinc in Alzheimer's disease. Cell
      2010;142:857-867.

[20] Wang Z, Wang B, Yang L, et al. Presynaptic and postsynaptic interaction of the amy-
      loid precursor protein promotes peripheral and central synaptogenesis. J Neurosci
      2009;29:10788-10801.

[21] Yang L, Wang B, Long C, Wu G, Zheng H. Increased asynchronous release and aber-
      rant calcium channel activation in amyloid precursor protein deficient neuromuscu-
      lar synapses. Neurosci 2007;149:768-778.

[22] Dinet V, An N, Ciccotosto GD, et al. APP involvement in retinogenesis of mice. Acta
      Neuropathol 2011;121:351-363.

[23] Ho T, Vessey KA, Cappai R, et al. Amyloid Precursor Protein Is Required for Normal Function of the Rod and Cone Pathways n the Mouse Retina. PLoS One 2012;7.

[24] Lee VM-Y, Goedert M, Trojanowski JQ. Neurodegenerative tauopathies. Annual Review of Neuroscience 2001;24:1121-1159.

[25] Spires-Jones TL, Stoothoff WH, de Calignon A, Jones PB, Hyman BT. Tau pathophysiology in neurodegeneration: a tangled ssue. Trends Neurosci 2009;32:150-159.

[26] Dawson HN, Ferreira A, Eyster MV, Ghoshal N, Binder LI, Vitek MP. Inhibition of neuronal maturation in primary hippocampal neurons from tau deficient mice. J Cell Sci 2001;114:1179-1187.

[27] Ittner LM, Ke YD, Delerue F, et al. Dendritic function of tau mediates amyloid-beta toxicity in Alzheimer's disease mouse models. Cell 2010;142:387-397.

[28] Hwang SC, Jhon DY, Bae YS, Kim JH, Rhee SG. Activation of phospholipase C-gamma by the concerted action of tau proteins and arachidonic acid. J Biol Chem 1996;271:18342-18349.

[29] Perez M, Santa-Maria I, Gomez de Barreda E, et al. Tau--an inhibitor of deacetylase HDAC6 function. J Neurochem 2009;109:1756-1766.

[30] Miao Y, Chen J, Zhang Q, Sun A. Deletion of tau attenuates heat shock-induced injury in cultured cortical neurons. J Neurosci Res 2010;88:102-110.

[31] Shahani N, Brandt R. Functions and malfunctions of the tau proteins. Cell Mol Life Sci 2002;59:1668-1680.

[32] Hong M, Zhukareva V, Vogelsberg-Ragaglia V, et al. Mutation-specific functional impairments in distinct tau isoforms of hereditary FTDP-17. Science 1998;282:1914-1917.

[33] Lieven CJ, Millet LE, Hoegger MJ, Levin LA. Induction of axon and dendrite formation during early RGC-5 cell differentiation. Exp Eye Res 2007;85:678-683.

[34] Nakayama T, Goshima Y, Misu Y, Kato T. Role of cdk5 and tau phosphorylation in heterotrimeric G protein-mediated retinal growth cone collapse. J Neurobiol 1999;41:326-339.

[35] Liu B, Rasool S, Yang Z, et al. Amyloid-peptide vaccinations reduce {beta}-amyloid plaques but exacerbate vascular deposition and inflammation in the retina of Alzheimer's transgenic mice. The American journal of pathology 2009;175:2099-2110.

[36] Nikolic M, Dudek H, Kwon YT, Ramos YF, Tsai LH. The cdk5/p35 kinase is essential for neurite outgrowth during neuronal differentiation. Genes Dev 1996;10:816-825.

[37] Arimura N, Inagaki N, Chihara K, et al. Phosphorylation of collapsin response mediator protein-2 by Rho-kinase. Evidence for two separate signaling pathways for growth cone collapse. J Bio Chem 2000;275:23973-23980.

[38] Cheng Q, Sasaki Y, Shoji M, et al. Cdk5/p35 and Rho-kinase mediate ephrin-A5-induced signaling in retinal ganglion cells. Mol Cel Neurosci 2003;24:632-645.

[39] Liu N, Cooper NG. The Ca2+/calmodulin-dependent protein kinase II-associated protein complex isolated from chicken retina. J Mol Neurosci 1996;7:1-12.

[40] Stamer K, Vogel R, Thies E, Mandelkow E, Mandelkow EM. Tau blocks traffic of organelles, neurofilaments, and APP vesicles n neurons and enhances oxidative stress. J Cell Bio 2002;156:1051-1063.

[41] Magnani E, Fan J, Gasparini L, et al. Interaction of tau protein with the dynactin complex. Embo J 2007;26:4546-4554.

[42] Cogan DG. Alzheimer syndromes. Am J Ophthalmol 1987;104:183-184.

[43] Katz B, Rimmer S, Iragui V, Katzman R. Abnormal pattern electroretinogram in Alzheimer's disease - evidence for retinal ganglion-cell degeneration. Ann Neurol 1989;26:221-225.

[44] Katz B, Rimmer S, Iragui V, Katzman R. Abnormal pattern electroretinogram in Alzheimer's disease: evidence for retinal ganglion cell degeneration? Ann Neurol 1989;26:221-225.

[45] Jackson GR, Owsley C. Visual dysfunction, neurodegenerative diseases, and aging. Neurol Clin 2003;21:709-728.

[46] Lee AG, Martin CO. Neuro-ophthalmic findings in the visual variant of Alzheimer's disease. Ophthalmol 2004;111:376-380.

[47] Cronin-Golomb A, Corkin S, Rizzo JF, Cohen J, Growdon JH, Banks KS. Visual dysfunction in Alzheimer's disease: relation to normal aging. Ann Neurol 1991;29:41-52.

[48] Mendez MF, Cherrier MM, Meadows RS. Depth perception in Alzheimer's disease. Percept Mot Skills 1996;83:987-995.

[49] Cronin-Golomb A. Vision in Alzheimer's disease. Gerontologist 1995;35:370-376.

[50] Gilmore GC, Whitehouse PJ. Contrast sensitivity in Alzheimer's disease: a 1-year longitudinal analysis. Optom Vis Sci 1995;72:83-91.

[51] Leuba G, Saini K. Pathology of subcortical visual centers in relation to cortical degeneration in Alzheimers-disease. Neuropath Applied Neurobiol 1995;21:410-422.

[52] Koronyo-Hamaoui M, Koronyo Y, Ljubimov AV, et al. Identification of amyloid plaques in retinas from Alzheimer's patients and noninvasive in vivo optical imaging of retinal plaques in a mouse model. Neuroimage 2011;54S1:S204-S217.

[53] Paquet C, Boissonnot M, Roger F, Dighiero P, Gil R, Hugon J. Abnormal retinal thickness in patients with mild cognitive mpairment and Alzheimer's disease. Neurosci Lett 2007;420:97-99.

[54] Berisha F, Feke GT, Trempe CL, McMeel JW, Schepens CL. Retinal abnormalities in early Alzheimer's disease. Investigative ophthalmology & visual science 2007;48:2285-2289.

[55] Iseri PK, Altinas O, Tokay T, Yuksel N. Relationship between cognitive impairment and retinal morphological and visual functional abnormalities in Alzheimer disease. J Neuroophthalmol 2006;26:18-24.

[56] Parisi V. Correlation between morphological and functional retinal impairment in patients affected by ocular hypertension, glaucoma, demyelinating optic neuritis and Alzheimer's disease. Semin Ophthalmol 2003;18:50-57.

[57] Valenti DA. Neuroimaging of retinal nerve fiber layer in AD using optical coherence tomography. Neurology 2007;69:1060.

[58] Danesh-Meyer HV, Birch H, Ku JY, Carroll S, Gamble G. Reduction of optic nerve fibers in patients with Alzheimer disease dentified by laser imaging. Neurol 2006;67:1852-1854.

[59] Hinton DR, Sadun AA, Blanks JC, Miller CA. Optic-nerve degeneration in Alzheimer's disease. N Engl J Med 1986;315:485-487.

[60] Sadun AA, Bassi CJ. Optic nerve damage in Alzheimer's disease. Ophthalmology 1990;97:9-17.

[61] Foster PJ, Buhrmann R, Quigley HA, Johnson GJ. The definition and classification of glaucoma in prevalence surveys. Bri J Ophthalmol 2002;86:238-242.

[62] Quigley HA. Glaucoma. Lancet 2011;377:1367-1377.

[63] Parisi V, Restuccia R, Fattapposta F, Mina C, Bucci MG, Pierelli F. Morphological and functional retinal impairment in Alzheimer's disease patients. Clin Neurophysiol 2001;112:1860-1867.

[64] Nesher R, Trick GL. The pattern electroretinogram in retinal and optic-nerve disease - a quantitative comparison of the pattern of visual dysfunction. Doc Ophthalmol 1991;77:225-235.

[65] McKinnon SJ, Lehman DM, Kerrigan-Baumrind LA, et al. Caspase activation and amyloid precursor protein cleavage in rat ocular hypertension. Invest Ophthalmol Vis Sci 2002;43:1077-1087.

[66] Yin H, Chen L, Chen X, Liu X. Soluble amyloid beta oligomers may contribute to apoptosis of retinal ganglion cells in glaucoma. Med Hypotheses 2008;71:77-80.

[67] Bayer AU, Ferrari F, Erb C. High occurrence rate of glaucoma among patients with Alzheimer's disease. Eur Neurol 2002;47:165-168.

[68] Price DL, Tanzi RE, Borchelt DR, Sisodia SS. Alzheimer's disease: genetic studies and transgenic models. Annu Rev Genet 1998;32:461-493.

[69] Chiu K, Chan TF, Wu A, Leung IYP, So KF, Chang RCC. Neurodegeneration of the retina in mouse models of Alzheimer's disease: what can we learn from the retina? Age 2012;34:633-649.

[70] Arendash GW, Lewis J, Leighty RE, et al. Multi-metric behavioral comparison of APPsw and P301L models for Alzheimer's disease: linkage of poorer cognitive performance to tau pathology in forebrain. Brain Res 2004;1012:29-41.

[71] Wostyn P, Audenaert K, De Deyn PP. Alzheimer's disease-related changes in diseases characterized by elevation of ntracranial or intraocular pressure. Clin Neurol Neurosurg 2008;110:101-109.

[72] Muyllaert D, Kremer A, Jaworski T, et al. Glycogen synthase kinase-3beta, or a link between amyloid and tau pathology? Genes Brain Behav 2008;7 Suppl 1:57-66.

[73] Liu B, Rasool S, Yang Z, et al. Amyloid-peptide vaccinations reduce {beta}-amyloid plaques but exacerbate vascular deposition and inflammation in the retina of Alzheimer's transgenic mice. Am J Pathol 2009;175:2099-2110.

[74] Cordeiro MF, Guo L, Coxon KM, et al. Imaging multiple phases of neurodegeneration: a novel approach to assessing cell death n vivo. Cell Death and Dis 2010;1:e3.

[75] Dutescu RM, Li QX, Crowston J, Masters CL, Baird PN, Culvenor JG. Amyloid precursor protein processing and retinal pathology in mouse models of Alzheimer's disease. Graefes Archive for Clinical and Experimental Ophthalmology 2009;247:1213-1221.

[76] Dutescu RM, Li QX, Crowston J, Masters CL, Baird PN, Culvenor JG. Amyloid precursor protein processing and retinal pathology in mouse models of Alzheimer's disease. Graefes Arch Clin Exp Ophthalmol 2009;247:1213-1221.

[77] Perez SE, Lumayag S, Kovacs B, Mufson EJ, Xu S. Beta-amyloid deposition and functional impairment in the retina of the APPswe/PS1DeltaE9 transgenic mouse model of Alzheimer's disease. Invest Ophthalmol Vis Sci 2009;50:793-800.

[78] Gasparini L, Crowther RA, Martin KR, et al. Tau inclusions in retinal ganglion cells of human P301S tau transgenic mice: effects on axonal viability. Neurobio aging 2011;32:419-433.

[79] Oddo S, Caccamo A, Shepherd JD, et al. Triple-transgenic model of Alzheimer's disease with plaques and tangles: intracellular Abeta and synaptic dysfunction. Neuron 2003;39:409-421.

[80] Bull ND, Guidi A, Goedert M, Martin KR, Spillantini MG. Reduced Axonal Transport and Increased Excitotoxic Retinal Ganglion Cell Degeneration in Mice Transgenic for Human Mutant P301S Tau. PLoS One 2012;7.

[81] Guo L, Salt TE, Luong V, et al. Targeting amyloid-beta in glaucoma treatment. Proc Natl Acad Sci U S A 2007;104:13444-13449.

[82] Goldblum D, Kipfer-Kauer A, Sarra GM, Wolf S, Frueh BE. Distribution of amyloid precursor protein and amyloid-beta mmunoreactivity in DBA/2J glaucomatous mouse retinas. Invest Ophthalmol Vis Sci 2007;48:5085-5090.

[83] Kipfer-Kauer A, McKinnon SJ, Frueh BE, Goldblum D. Distribution of Amyloid Precursor Protein and Amyloid-beta in Ocular Hypertensive C57BL/6 Mouse Eyes. Cur Eye Res 2010;35:828-834.

[84] Hung CH, Ho YS, Chang RCC. Modulation of mitochondrial calcium as a pharmacological target for Alzheimer's disease. Ageing Res Rev 2010;9:447-456.

[85] Saotome M, Safiulina D, Szabadkai G, et al. Bidirectional Ca2+-dependent control of mitochondrial dynamics by the Miro GTPase. Proc Natl Acad Sci U S A 2008;105:20728-20733.

[86] Liu X, Hajnoczky G. Ca2+-dependent regulation of mitochondrial dynamics by the Miro-Milton complex. Int J Biochem Cell Biol 2009;41:1972-1976.

[87] Allen B, Ingram E, Takao M, et al. Abundant tau filaments and nonapoptotic neurodegeneration in transgenic mice expressing human P301S tau protein. J Neurosci 2002;22:9340-9351.

[88] Wang X, Su B, Lee HG, et al. Impaired balance of mitochondrial fission and fusion in Alzheimer's disease. J Neurosci 2009;29:9090-9103.

[89] Carelli V, Ross-Cisneros FN, Sadun AA. Mitochondrial dysfunction as a cause of optic neuropathies. Prog Retin Eye Res 2004;23:53-89.

[90] Ju WK, Liu Q, Kim KY, et al. Elevated hydrostatic pressure triggers mitochondrial fission and decreases cellular ATP in differentiated RGC-5 cells. Invest Ophthalmol Vis Sci 2007;48:2145-2151.

[91] Abu-Amero KK, Morales J, Bosley TM. Mitochondrial Abnormalities in Patients with Primary Open-Angle Glaucoma. Investigative Ophthalmology & Visual Science 2006;47:2533-2541.

[92] Neroev VV, Archipova MM, Bakeeva LE, et al. Mitochondria-targeted plastoquinone derivatives as tools to interrupt execution of the aging program. 4. Age-related eye disease. SkQ1 returns vision to blind animals. Biochemistry (Mosc) 2008.

[93] Leger F, Fernagut PO, Canron MH, et al. Protein aggregation in the aging retina. J Neuropath Exp Neurol 2011;70:63-68.

[94] Gupta N, Fong J, Ang LC, Yucel YH. Retinal tau pathology in human glaucomas. Can J Ophthalmol 2008;43:53-60.

[95] Oka T, Tamada Y, Nakajima E, Shearer TR, Azuma M. Presence of calpain-induced proteolysis in retinal degeneration and dysfunction in a rat model of acute ocular hypertension. J Neurosci Res 2006;83:1342-1351.

[96]   Tamada Y, Nakajima E, Nakajima T, Shearer TR, Azuma M. Proteolysis of neuronal cytoskeletal proteins by calpain contributes to rat retinal cell death induced by hypoxia. Brain Res 2005;1050:148-155.

[97]   Guo L, Duggan J, Cordeiro MF. Alzheimer's disease and retinal neurodegeneration. Curr Alzheimer Res 2010;7:3-14.

[98]   Kong GY, Van Bergen NJ, Trounce IA, Crowston JG. Mitochondrial dysfunction and glaucoma. J Glaucoma 2009;18:93-100.

[99]   Chang RCC, Suen KC, Ma CH, Elyaman W, Ng HK, Hugon J. Involvement of double-stranded RNA-dependent protein kinase and phosphorylation of eukaryotic initiation factor-2 alpha in neuronal degeneration. Journal of Neurochemistry 2002a; 83:1215-1225.

[100] Chang RCC, Wong AKY, Ng HK, Hugon J. Phosphorylation of eukaryotic initiation factor-2 alpha (eIF2 alpha) is associated with neuronal degeneration in Alzheimer's disease. Neuroreport 2002b;13:2429-2432.

[101] Suen KC, Yu MS, So KF, Chang RCC, Hugon J. Upstream signaling pathways leading to the activation of double-stranded RNA-dependent serine/threonine protein kinase in {beta}-amyloid peptide neurotoxicity. J Bio Chem 2003;278:49819-49827.

[102] Shimazawa M, Ito Y, Inokuchi Y, Hara H. Involvement of Double-Stranded RNA-Dependent Protein Kinase in ER Stress-Induced Retinal Neuron Damage. Invest Ophthalmol Vis Sci 2007;48:3729-3736.

[103] Chan HC, Chang RCC, Koon-Ching Ip A, et al. Neuroprotective effects of Lycium barbarum Lynn on protecting retinal ganglion cells in an ocular hypertension model of glaucoma. Exp Neurol 2007;203:269-273.

[104] Yu MS, Lai CS, Ho YS, et al. Characterization of the effects of anti-aging medicine Fructus lycii on beta-amyloid peptide neurotoxicity. Int J Mol Med 2007;20:261-268.

[105] Ho YS, Yu MS, Yang XF, So KF, Yuen WH, Chang RCC. Neuroprotective Effects of Polysaccharides from Wolfberry, the Fruits of Lycium barbarum, Against Homocysteine-induced Toxicity in Rat Cortical Neurons. J Alzheimers Dis 2009.

[106] Ho YS, Yu MS, Yik SY, So KF, Yuen WH, Chang RCC. Polysaccharides from wolfberry antagonizes glutamate excitotoxicity in rat cortical neurons. Cell Mol Neurobiol 2009;29:1233-1244.

[107] Yu MS, Ho YS, So KF, Yuen WH, Chang RCC. Cytoprotective effects of Lycium barbarum against reducing stress on endoplasmic reticulum. Int J Mol Med 2006;17:1157-1161.

[108] Chiu K, Chan HC, Yeung SC, et al. Erratum: Modulation of microglia by Wolfberry on the survival of retinal ganglion cells in a rat ocular hypertension model. J Ocul Biol Dis Infor 2009;2:127-136.

[109] Chiu K, Zhou Y, Yeung SC, et al. Up-regulation of crystallins is involved in the neuroprotective effect of wolfberry on survival of retinal ganglion cells in rat ocular hypertension model. J Cell Biochem 2010;110:311-320.

[110] Garcia-Alloza M, Robbins EM, Zhang-Nunes SX, et al. Characterization of amyloid deposition in the APPswe/PS1dE9 mouse model of Alzheimer disease. Neurobiol Dis 2006;24:516-524.

[111] Garcia-Alloza M, Borrelli LA, Rozkalne A, Hyman BT, Bacskai BJ. Curcumin labels amyloid pathology in vivo, disrupts existing plaques, and partially restores distorted neurites in an Alzheimer mouse model. J Neurochem 2007;102:1095-1104.

[112] Yang F, Lim GP, Begum AN, et al. Curcumin Inhibits Formation of Amyloid β Oligomers and Fibrils, Binds Plaques, and Reduces Amyloid in Vivo. J Biol Chem 2005;280:5892-5901.

[113] Baum L, Lam CWK, Cheung SK-K, et al. Six-Month Randomized, Placebo-Controlled, Double-Blind, Pilot Clinical Trial of Curcumin in Patients With Alzheimer Disease. J Clin Psych 2008;28:110-113

[114] Hintersteiner M, Enz A, Frey P, et al. In vivo detection of amyloid-beta deposits by near-infrared imaging using an oxazine-derivative probe. Nat Biotechnol 2005;23:577-583.

[115] Nakada T, Matsuzawa H, Igarashi H, Fujii Y, Kwee IL. In vivo visualization of senile-plaque-like pathology in Alzheimer's disease patients by MR microscopy on a 7T system. J Neuroimaging 2008;18:125-129.

Chapter 7

Minimally Invasive Glaucoma Surgery – Strategies for Success

Daljit Singh

Additional information is available at the end of the chapter

1. Introduction

The aim of glaucoma surgery is to drain the internal reservoir of aqueous in such a manner that the inside head pressure remains within normal limits.The conventional and alternative pathways have been well known for decades - the anterior route that goes through the canal of Schlemm and the posterior route which is called "uveo-scleral outflow". While the former route has been studied and discussed thoroughly for over a century, the latter mechanism has been discovered only recently and is talked about more as a functional rather than an anatomical entity. When the natural drainage mechanisms get stressed for any reason, the intra ocular pressure rises proportionately. The dearth of knowledge about the involvement of an extensive lymphatic channel system in aqueous drainage, has unwittingly encouraged the surgeons to perform dissections on the sclera with a rather large footprint. Bipolar cautery is used with impunity for the same reason. We shall now discuss the lymphatic channel system.

2. Lymphatics

Without a shadow of doubt, it has been proved that the conjunctival lymphatics do exist [1,12,17,22,23,24]. Every glaucoma surgeon should verify it with his own eyes. Under high magnification of a slit lamp microscope, the lymphatics are visible at the limbus, especially if there is some pigment. Pigment highlights the lymphatics. They stand out in cases of sub-conjunctival haemorhage as a result of trauma, accidental or surgical. The blood is drained through the lymphatics. The network of lymphatics can be charted by injecting tyrpan blue at the limbus. Injection of the dye in the sclera demonstrates scleral channels as well as their continuity with the sub-conjunctival lymphatics. Yeni et al [28] have demonstrated the presence of lymphatics in the ciliary body. It becomes obvious that uveoscleral outflow is actually a channel based aqueous pathway. No lymphatics can be demonstrated in the areas of subconjunctival scarring. All glaucoma surgeons need to be aware of the lymphatics.

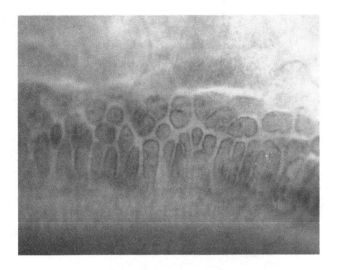

Figure 1. Limbal lymphatics.They enter the cornea singly, but anastomose proximally and join the conjunctival lymphatic network.The presence of pigment at the limbus makes the lymphatics prominent.

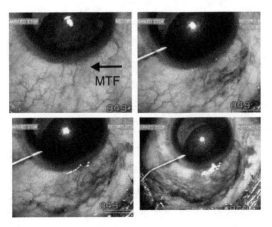

Figure 2. Microtrack filtration was done one day earlier to control glaucoma after blunt injury.Before removing dislocated lens, trypan blue was injected to chart lymphatics of conjunctva.

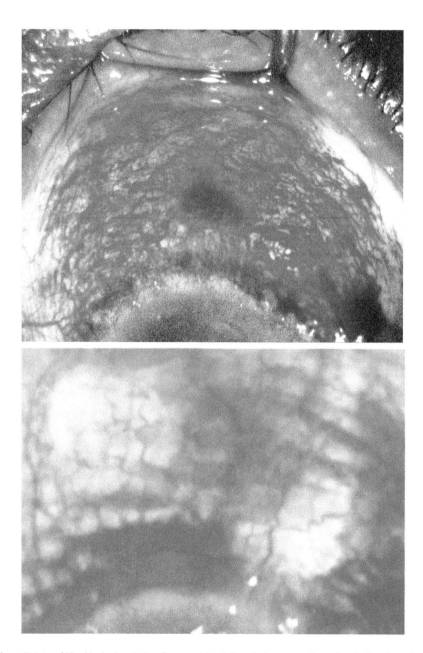

Figure 3. Entry of blood in the lymphatics after an unintended surgical trauma to the conjunctiva. Two hours later, most of the blood had migrated in to the conjunctival lymphatics.

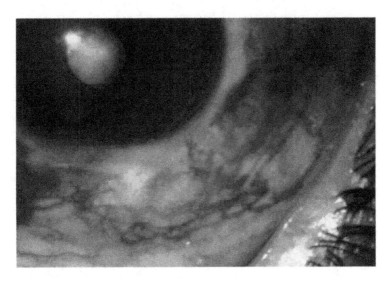

Figure 4. A failed case of trabeculectomy. Dye injection fails to show lymphatics in the totally scarred central area. The seen lymphatics are thin and have a disturbed pattern.

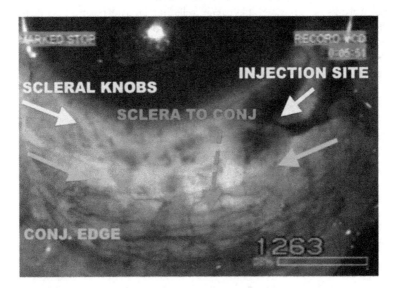

Figure 5. It demonstrates the intrascleral movement of injected trypan blue along the limbus where it ends in knobs. The proximal movement of the dye through the sclera enters the subconjunctival lymphatics, proving that conjunctival and scleral channels are one system.

Anatomy is the basis of physiology. The lymphatics drain the extracellular fluid, one that comes out of the arterial ends of the capillaries, the leakage from the aqueous veins and the uveoscleral outflow. The drainage occurs all around the limbus. When a filtration surgery is performed, there is a huge local outflow, which can be handled only by the flood drain like function of the lymphatics. Their sizes and capabilities match the changing needs after filtration surgery.

The techniques of glaucoma surgery are limited by the tools that are employed to achieve them. For the last one century,the tools are basically the same - forceps, scissors, knife and cautery. Only they are now finer and sharper. Excellent magnification and coaxial light are recent helps for the surgeon. Tissues are cut and dissected in layers, which are sutured back, after making a large opening in to the anterior chamber. Tissue reaction and scarring is a serious concern to manage/prevent which anti-mitotics are used during and often post-surgery.

The arrival of a radically new surgical tool, Fugo blade, providing plasma energy on the tip of a filament has remained largely un-noticed or un-understood outside the United States and even less actually used.

2.1. What is Fugo blade ?

Fugo blade [3,4,8,9,13,14,15,16,17,26,27] produces "laser like plasma" on the operating blunt metal tip. It works on 4 rechargeable battery cells.Numerous glaucoma operations can be done after one charge. Cut power and intensity can be adjusted from the console. How does it function ? It focusses electromagnetic energy to the operating tip.The energy is pre-tuned to the tissues and is transferred by resonance. The moment the activated tip touches the tissues, the energy gets transferred to the tissue molecules, which go to higher energy levels, become unstable and explode, just as happens with excimer laser when it acts on the cornea.A plume with aromatic smell is produced.The molecules/tissues split in the path of incision/ablation.The incisions are bloodless, since the small blood vessels are also removed from the path of incision.It is possible to ablate surfaces and create channels/tracks in simple and efficient manner.

The width of the cutting plasma coating on the operating tip can be varied from "power" adjustment- 25, 50 or 75 microns.The intensity can be varied from 1 to 10 from the second knob.

Fugo blade application in glaucoma surgery raises a dilemma. You cannot make the traditional surgery any better with it. So why use it? That it opens newer ways to do glaucoma surgery is not yet attractive, because the new techniques have not yet been approved and advocated by the stalwarts in the field. That in stead of dissecting in layers, you can tap the aqueous chambers through direct track formation seems frightening, since it breaks the five decades old taboo by not making a "guarding scleral flap". The scleral flap in trabeculectomy might help prevent over-filtration, but the prevention of infection always rests upon healthy conjunctiva.

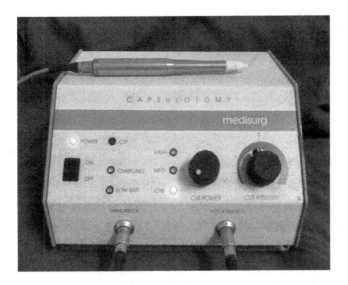

Figure 6. Fugo blade console, hand piece and the disposable operating tip.One connection goes to the hand-piece and the other to the foot-switch. The left knob is for cut power and the right for intensity. Manufacturer: Medisurg Ltd. c/o Richard J. Fugo. 100 West Fornance St. The Fugo Building. Norristown, Pa 19401.USA

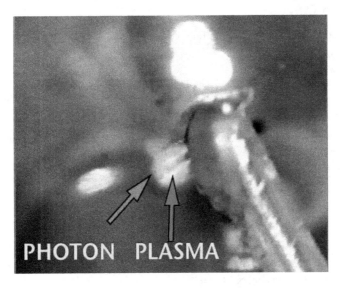

Figure 7. High magnification photograph of activated Fugo blade tip showing yellow plasma coating (cutting) around the metal filament and the orange photonic cloud (non cutting).

In short, lack of awareness about the lymphatic network that drains the aqueous normally and that works like flood drains after filtration surgery, and the failure to appreciate new possibilities of glaucoma surgery that are opened up with Fugo plasma blade, keeps the modern glaucoma surgery where it is - essentially a standstill.

2.2. Minimally invasive glaucoma surgery

Trabeculectomy or its modification remains the operation of choice for most surgeons. Non perforating filtration under a scleral flap and glaucoma valve are other choices. Every operation makes a fairly large foot print on the sclera and inevitably destroys the lymphatics in the surgical field. This happens because the surgery involves making flaps of the tissues. A "guarded flap" is a necessity for making a rather large trabeculectomy opening at the limbus.

2.3. Transciliary Filtration (TCF)

Fugo blade allows the making of a filtration track (TCF) in to the posterior chamber.There is no other tool that has this capability. The filtration track goes through the sclera and the ciliary body to reach the posterior chamber[2,5,6,7,10,17,19,21,23]. TCF may be done after making a fornix or limbus based conjunctival flap, which involves some/considerable trauma. Transconjunctival(TC) TCF minimizes surgical trauma. TCF prevents anterior chamber problems like a shallow or flat anterior chamber and hyphaema. No iridectomy is done in this operation.

In all the operations described below, subconjunctival anaesthesia is given.

The steps of TCTCF are as follows:

1. The posterior edge of the surgical limbus is visible through the conjunctiva. It lies over the the anterior corneo-scleral trabeculae. A point is chosen 1.5 mm posterior to it.This point is pressed with the blunt tip of a forceps to leave a mark on the sclera.

2. A 300 micron or 500 micron Fugo blade tip is chosen to be used at high power and intensity. The conjunctiva is pushed towards the limbus with a blunt sapphire knife till it reaches the marked point on the sclera.

3. The activated Fugo blade is passed through the conjunctiva, the sclera and the ciliary body to reach the posterior chamber. The track may be made in one step or a series of small steps progressively taking the track to the posterior chamber. The end point shows as aqueous drainage. Nothing further needs to be done.

4. 0.1 ml to 0.2 ml of Mitomycin C (MMC) 0.01 % or 0.02 % is deposited under the conjunctiva. The conjunctival opening is sutured.

An anteriorly misdirected track can open in to the anterior chamber and posterior misdirection can lead to the vitreous show/prolapse.

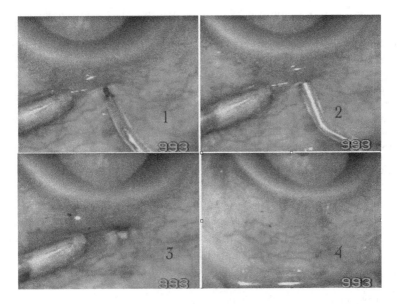

Figure 8. in a case of phakomorphic glaucoma.The conjunctiva is pushed towards the limbus up to a pre-determined point.Fugo blade tip passes through the conjunctiva, the sclera and the ciliary body to drain the posterior chamber.

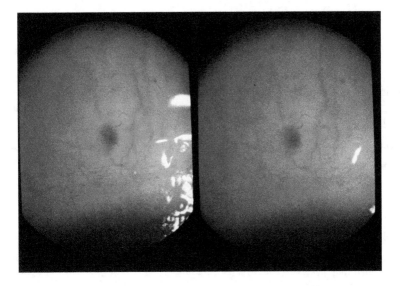

Figure 9. TCTCF with a 500 micron Fugo blade tip in a case of neovascular glaucoma, one day after surgery

TCTCF is the least traumatic way to drain the posterior chamber. It is most useful in cases of acute congestive glaucoma, phakomorphic glaucoma and neovascular glaucoma. The last group of cases show vascularization of the iris and the angle, but there are no such changes over the ciliary body. TCTCF can be done in any case with a normal posterior chamber.

TCTCF does pass through the tenon capsule, the thickness of the sclera and the highly vascular ciliary body, which is a trauma, howsoever slight it may be.

The following film depicts TCTCF in a difficult case of neovascular glaucoma. There was extensive scarring around the limbus. TCTCF was done by approaching the posterior chamber, from beyond the scarred area.

http://www.youtube.com/watch?v=uO57F9gdTU4

TCTCF is handy to treat cases of phakomorphic glaucoma that has lasted for many days or weeks (a common happening in the third world).There is a vicious cycle of the swollen cataract raising IOP and the raised IOP pushing more fluid in to the swollen lens. The moment the posterior chamber drainage starts, there is an improvement in the depth of the anterior chamber. Over days one can see a diminution in the thickness of the intumescent cataract.

The following film shows TCTCF in a case of phakomorphic glaucoma:

http://www.youtube.com/watch?v=wSWrIr7Jesc

Now we turn our attention to anterior chamber filtration and look at the opportunities that it offers for minimally traumatic filtration surgery.

2.4. Microtrack Filtration

Microtrack Filtration (MTF) makes a track between the anterior chamber and the anterior most area of subconjunctival space[17,20,25]. If a filtering track between 100 micron to 250 micron could be sustained without internal block and outer scarring, and the aqueous kept seeping out and getting drained by the network of lymphatics, the problem of glaucoma is as good as solved. Easier said than done.Even a microtrack creates a few hurdles that need to be crossed.

Let us first describe the technique of Microtrack Filtration. The steps of surgery are as follows:

1. Anaesthesia: Facial block and subconjunctival injection of lignocaine in adults. General anesthesia in children.

2. Eyeball fixation: An episcleral suture is passed close to the nasal limbus and the eye turned down.

3. Making an opening in the conjunctiva close to the 10 O' clock limbus with a Fugo blade 100 micron tip.

4. Through this hole, 0.1 to 0.2 ml of mitomycin C (MMC) 0.01 % or 0.02 %, is injected under the conjunctiva with a 30 gauge cannula, to raise a bleb at the upper limbus.

5. A pocket incision is made in the anterior chamber with a 0.75 mm diamond knife close to the limbus. Depending upon the surgical plan of peripheral iridectomy, it may be made in line with 3 O' clock, 9 O' clock or 12 O' clock.

6. Pilocarpine or carbachol is injected in the anterior chamber to contract the pupil.

7. Two or three iridotomies are made in the iris periphery, with the help of a 100 micron Fugo blade tip.The iris is touched with the tip and then activated with the highest energy-an opening gets made instantly. Pigment from the posterior pigment epithelium raises a small cloud. The anterior chamber is irrigated with a 30 gauge cannula. It is also passed through the iridotomies to make sure they are patent.

8. A 1.5 mm 100 micron Fugo blade tip is passed through 12 O' clock conjunctiva about 7-8 mm from the limbus, with the lowest energy. It is then pushed under the ballooned/raised conjunctiva in un-activated form, to reach the limbus.When the tip reaches the limbus/desired point, its location is clearly visualized.

9. The tip is raised by about 30 degrees, while its point remains engaged at the limbus,close to, but slightly away from the attachment of conjunctiva.We wish to avoid conjunctival puncture at the time of microtrack formation.

10. The track making is the next step. The machine has been set at the desired power and intensity levels. The point of the tip is lightly pushing the limbal tissues, when it is activated. In a fraction of a second,it passes through the limbus in to the anterior chamber.As the tip is withdrawn, the aqueous follows, raising an enlarging bleb. A track about 250 micron wide, gets formed anterior to the corneo-scleral trabeculae.

11. Air is injected to deepen the anterior chamber.

12. Sodium hyaluronate (NaHa) in the anterior chamber is optional.It also helps to keep the anterior chamber deep.

Application of MTF:

Any patient with a healthy/virgin perilimbal conjunctiva and an intact anterior chamber is suitable for this operation. It can be used at any age. The surgical trauma is minimal, compared to all other available manual or laser procedures.

Here are some films on MTF:

http://www.youtube.com/watch?v=C5pHb2JfmaA

MTF in a case of buphthalmos is shown here:

http://www.youtube.com/watch?v=XKQ9-JnBx9I

MTF in a case of keratouveitis is shown here:

http://www.youtube.com/watch?v=C5pHb2JfmaA

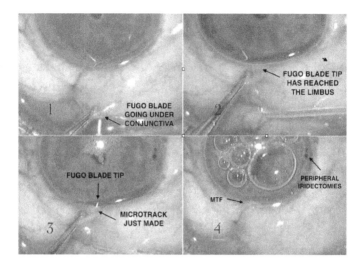

Figure 10. Fugo blade tip is passed through the ballooned conjunctiva about 7 mm from the limbus.It is then pushed to the limbus in un-activated form. Activation of the tip instantly makes MTF track.

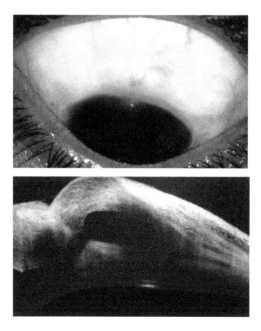

Figure 11. Microtrack filtration, one year after surgery. OCT shows MTF track.

Postoperative course and management:

In the beginning the normal subconjunctival tissues offer little resistance to the outward flow of the aqueous. This little resistance is what keeps the anterior chamber formed, even though it is on the shallower side. We need to keep the iris away from the internal opening of the track. Therefore from day one the pupil is kept contracted by pilocarpine 2% three times a day.I firmly believe that lymphatics play a definite role in offering resistance to aqueous outflow. Initially they act as flood drains, but the outflow is so excessive that a big conjunctival bleb is formed. Later the initial rush of aqueous is over. Then sets in a balance between the out going aqueous and the tissue resistance,at least a part of which is resistance from the lymphatics.The anterior chamber begins to deepen. If it deepens too fast, and the bleb begins to dry up, it is a sign of a partial or complete closure of internal opening by the iris which needs early correction. If the block is complete, the pressure goes high and the patient experiences pain and reduction of vision. The tiny internal blockage with iris shuts down the system. The fluid filled subconjunctival tissues start shrinking and become capable of greater resistance. The internal block is opened with a shot of Yag laser. Once the filtration restarts, the chances of its second time failure are much reduced. If the internal block is not opened for many days and weeks, the external opening also gets closed by healing process.Healing starts when fluid movement stops. One to two days of internal closure does not cause irreversible damage to the filtration track.In cases where cross-linked NaHa (Healaflow) has been used over the external opening track,the fluid movement has been restored after a week or even longer. During these crucial days the patient takes oral diamox and local pilocarpine drops.The moment the tiny piece of iris is detached with a shot of YAG laser, the filtration starts and conjunctival bleb forms.

It is thus clear that the first 3-4 weeks after surgery need very careful watch both by the surgeon and the patient. The vigilance is relaxed but not given up altogether after that. A regular follow up on a monthly or two monthly basis is a must for every glaucoma operated case.

In one recent report (Roy et al 2012) on Deep Sclerectomy in which Healaflow (cross linked sodium hyaluronate)had been used as adjunct, a sizable percentage (38.2 %) of patients required needling to treat bleb failure and encysted blebs. Nearly half (47.3 %) the patients required Nd:YAG laser goniopuncture.

After MTF procedure, there is no scope/necessity for a needling procedure. A bleb leakage never occurs, since a conjunctival flap is not made. The only intervention required/possible is a shot of Nd:YAG laser to disengage the iris if it sticks to the internal opening. If filtration is tardy and the pressure does not come below 20 mm, a combination of timolol and pilocarpine is started. The other medicine is the costlier latanoprost. If that too is ineffective or the patient feels the burden of cost, a re-operation is done. A re-operation is easy, since most of the conjunctiva along with lymphatics is intact.Failure is not an option, since a way can always be found to create a new filtration track.

Film: drainage of suprachoroidal fluid.

http://www.youtube.com/watch?v=M35h7JShnqc

Variations in Microtrack Filtration:

MMC may be deposited under the conjunctiva either at the beginning of surgery or at the end of it. We have ample photographic and OCT evidence that the lymphatics are not damaged by the concentrations used.

A side port incision serves many purposes - to make PI, to inject carbachol or NaHa. The last one is useful if more than one MTF tracks are planned. NaHa does not let the anterior chamber collapse, which allows a second or even a third MTF.

In some situations, especially repeat failures by any kind of technique, accompanied by subconjunctival scarring, it may be necessary to make a wider track up to 500 micron (300 micron tip at highest energy setting). In a case of perilimbal scar formation, the track formation is started proximal to the scar and a longish track is made through the sclera and limbus in to the anterior chamber.

Pre-tenon MTF:

The tenon capsule gets attached to the limbus, proximal to the attachment of the conjunctiva. Thus there is a potential subconjunctival space distal to the tenon attachment. This pretenon subconjunctival space can be approached to produce a somewhat tangential filtration track at the limbus. A film of this procedure can be see here:

http://www.youtube.com/watch?v=TXAw6tXPDfE&feature=endscreen

2.5. Choroidal detachment

Hypotony is the probable cause of choroidal detachment. There are greater chances of hypotony In aphakes,vitrectomized eyes, trauma, buphthalmos and high myopia cases.It may start soon after surgery or during the first 2 postoperative days. In some cases there is severe pain at the start. Fundus examination and b-scan reveal choroidal detachment - from slight to kissing choroidals. The situation is watched for a week, after which the suprachoroidal fluid is drained.

The steps of operation are as follows:

The conjunctiva is pushed towards the limbus from a distance of about 8 mm to a distance of 4-5 mm, with a blunt sapphire knife. A 100 micron Fugo blade tip is used to incise the conjunctiva, tenon capsule and the sclera, till supra-choroidal fluid starts draining. When sufficient fluid has drained, air is injected in the anterior chamber. No attempt is made to suture the scleral incision.The tenon capsule and the conjunctiva retract to normal. A couple of sutures are applied to the conjunctival incision.

Film: drainage of suprachoroidal fluid.

http://www.youtube.com/watch?v=M35h7JShnqc

Strategies to improve results with Microtrack Filtration

The strategies are based on the knowledge that the out coming aqueous is drained by the conjunctival lymphatics.Also on the observation that in the beginning the aqueous outflow is excessive and can sometimes cause excessive shallowing of the anterior chamber, leading to internal closure by the iris.

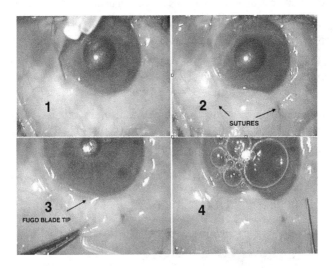

Figure 12. The ballooned conjunctiva is tied vertically on either side of 12 O' clock.Fugo blade is passed under the conjunctiva, taken to the limbus and MTF track made.A bleb gets formed.Air is injected in to the anterior chamber.

2.6. Tying the lymphatics

On either side of the proposed site of MTF, the conjunctiva is tied like a sheaf with a 10 zero suture. This ties the subconjunctival lymphatics too.

The steps of operation are as follows:

1. Making a hole in the conjunctiva close to the limbus of 10' O clock.

2. Injecting MMC 0.01%, 0.02 % through a 30 gauge cannula, to raise the conjunctiva widely, between 11 and 1 O' clock.

3. A suture is tied at 1 O' clock, starting near the limbus and getting out of the conjunctiva, three or four mm proximally. The bite catches the subconjunctival lymphatics along with the conjunctiva. The suture may be 10 zero prolene or 30 micron steel.It may be tied loosely with the intention of removing it after a few days. Or it may be tied fast, the intention being to leave the suture permanently. The second suture is tied at 11 O' clock. The conjunctiva gets raised between the two sutures.

4. A 0.75 mm corneal pocket incision is made close to the limbus, through which two iridotomies are made with a 2 mm long 100 micron Fugo blade tip. Highest energy is given to the tip to do iridotomy.

5. Anterior chamber is irrigated with a 30 gauge cannula. It is also used to verify the patency of iridotomies.

6. Microtrack filtration is done as usual. The raised conjunctiva only makes the job easier.

7. Air or NaHa or both are injected in the anterior chamber, through the pocket incision. NaHa can also be placed under the conjunctiva, between the two sutures.

The shape and the size of the filtration bleb is determined by the sutures.I call it a 'designer bleb'. The purpose is to restrict the outflow of aqueous, which reduces the tendency to shallowing of the anterior chamber, in the early postoperative period.

The resistance from the subconjunctival space between the sutures, can be further increased by putting cross linked NaHa (Healaflow) or collagen matrix (Ologen).

The purpose of every exercise is to control the depth of the anterior chamber.

Microtrack filtration, with two conjunctival sutures to restrain lymphatics is shown here:

http://www.youtube.com/watch?v=YYwalTIXQ0s

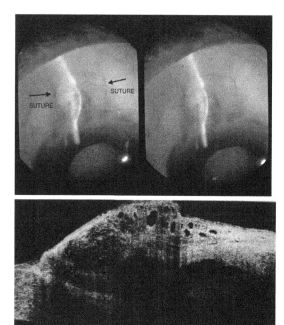

Figure 13. Bleb resulting from two conjunctival sutures, 5 months after surgery.The IOP is 12 mm from the initial 40 mm.The bleb has a good conjunctival cover. The proximal end of the bleb shows pleating. OCT shows the effect of two conjunctival sutures.There is a small kink. Lymphatics are also visible.

3. Intracameral suture

Intracameral sutures have been in use for a long time, mostly in relation to intraocular lens implants and trauma surgery. The tracks they make and the space they occupy are devoid of complications.

In connection with Microtrack filtration surgery, we thought of using intracameral sutures to prevent the iris from moving forward and closing the internal opening.The idea is to have a 10 zero polypropylene suture or a 30 micron stainless steel wire stretched in front of the iris periphery in the area of the MTF track.

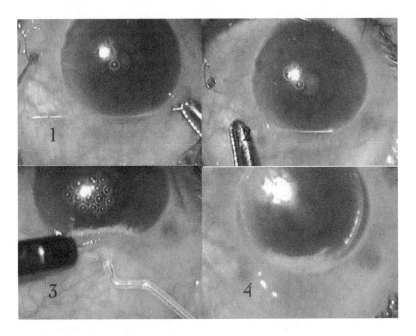

Figure 14. Transcameral suture is passed once towards the left and then it is returned to the right. The entry point is about 1 mm from the limbus in the sclera.Air is injected after MTF.

Steps of operation:

1. A small pocket incision in the cornea with a 0.75 mm diamond knife, at 3 O' clock or 12 O' clock.

2. The pupil is contracted with intracameral carbachol.

3. One two or three iridotomies are done in the periphery of the iris. The iridotomies are verified with a 30 gauge irrigation cannula.

4. A 1 cm + long straight needle carrying 10 zero prolene is passed through the upper part of the anterior chamber. The entry and the exit points are in the sclera, about 1 mm from the limbus. For leaving the suture permanently, the needle is returned parallel and close to the first route. The suture is tied and cut short and the knot buried.

5. A conjunctival hole is made at 10 O' clock close to the limbus. 0.1 to 0.2 ml of MMC 0.01% or 0.02 % is injected through a 30 gauge cannula, so as to raise a balloon. The fluid is spread out by the length of the cannula. Wait for 2 minutes.

6. MTF is done with a 100 micron Fugo blade tip is set at highest energy, which ablates a 250 micron track.

7. An air bubble is placed in the anterior chamber. NaHa can also be added to the anterior chamber to provide better stability.

MMC can be placed under the conjunctiva, either before or after doing MTF.

If a temporary intracameral suture is to be placed it is done as follows: The prolene carrying needle is passed through the anterior chamber, but is not pulled out on the other side, till MTF track has been made. The suture is tied over the limbus. The suture is stretched close and under the internal opening of the MTF track. This suture can be easily lifted and cut after 2-3 weeks, when the anterior chamber has become stabilized.Both variations of intracameral suture are seen in the following film:

http://www.youtube.com/watch?v=iNk_AsC-SEw

The procedure is somewhat cumbersome.

4. Viscoelastic resistance

The goal is to create resistance around the filtration track by injecting a viscoelastic material in the anterior chamber or subconjunctivally. NaHa is one such material. Its effectivity is difficult to perceive beyond 4-5 hours.

The other material is Healaflow- cross linked sodium hyaluronate, a material of high viscosity with an ability to stay in place for a long time and getting resorbed slowly. It has been used in all kinds of glaucoma operations as an adjunct since 2008.It has been used in the scleral space,under the scleral flap and under the conjunctiva. Healaflow is reticulated i.e. its architecture is like a network.This makes it a good space former and it has a long life span in situ.

The unique properties of Healaflow, make it particularly suitable as an adjunct in MTF. Under the conjunctiva, it is used as a "liquid cushion" against excessive flow during the first days and weeks after surgery. It is also our understanding that Healaflow presence under the conjunctiva shall retard the entry of aqueous in to the conjunctival lymphatics, create a sort of back pressure, that may prevent a flat anterior chamber. This reduces/prevents internal iris block.

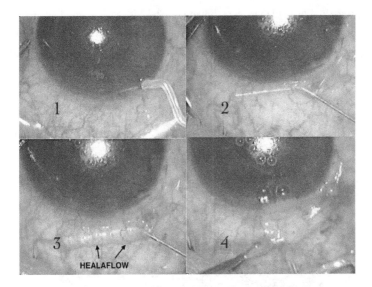

Figure 15. Peripheral iridotomy is made at 12 O' clock. Space is created along the limbus, in which Healaflow is deposited.MTF is done with 100 micron Fugo blade tip two times.The aqueous does not rush out since there is NaHa in the anterior chamber.

The steps of operation are as follows:

1. Making a conjunctival hole at 11 O'clock close to the limbus.

2. Raising a large bleb of MMC 0.01% or 0.02 % at the upper limbus.

3. Opening the anterior chamber with a pocket incision of 0.75 mm.

4. Contract the pupil with intracameral carbachol.

5. Making one or more peripheral iridotomies at 12 O'clock of the limbus.

6. Injecting NaHa in the anterior chamber close to the upper limbus.

7. Pushing away the subconjunctival fluid close to the limbus, with a cannula.

8. Through the existing conjunctival hole, Healaflow is injected along the upper limbus.it appears as a raised transparent strip along the limbus.The excess starts coming out through the conjunctival hole, which hole is closed with a single suture.

9. MTF is performed with a 100 micron Fugo blade glaucoma tip. With low energy it is passed through the conjunctiva about 7-8 mm from the limbus.It is then pushed towards the limbus unactivated, till the root of the conjunctiva is reached. The transparent raised Healaflow prominence improves the visibility of Fugo blade tip. Once the position of the tip clearly visualized, it is lifted at an angle of about 30 degrees, kept lightly pressed at the limbus as inactivated. The moment it is activated from the foot switch, it ablates a track

through the limbus in to the anterior chamber. There is only a slight flow of aqueous due to the presence of NaHa in the anterior chamber. The 100 micron Fugo blade tip if activated at high power, makes a precise 250 micron track.At medium power, the track shall be 200 microns.

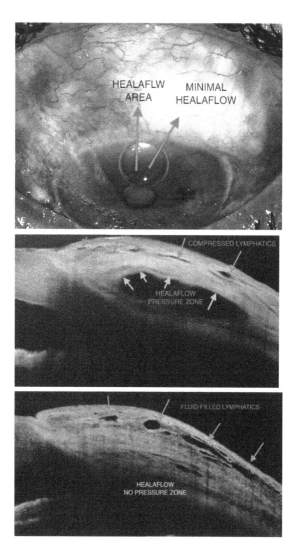

Figure 16. MTF with Healaflow 2 days after surgery. Healaflow compresses the overlying conjunctival lymphatics.The compression is maximum in the central area and minimum in the periphery

10. The conjunctival hole for MTF being only 150 micron, there is no need to apply a suture to it.

The use of NaHa inside the anterior chamber and Healaflow on the outside, provides excellent control on the flow of aqueous during surgery and for many hours and a few days after surgery. Even though NaHa shall disappear after some hours, Healaflow continues to exert the useful effect of a liquid cushion from the outside.

OCT done in the early postoperative days shows a dome of conjunctiva raised by Healaflow. The dome soon flattens out, after which it is difficult to discern clearly the location of Healaflow. For any dark slit like appearance, we can presume it to be that.

Conjunctival lymphatics act as flood drains for the aqueous and blood under the conjunctiva.Huge quantities of blood can be removed from the field quite efficiently. We have found that subconjunctival silicone oil is not taken away by the lymphatics. We do not know if Healaflow finally gets drained by lymphatics or it gets broken by the natural enzymes.

For delivering a precise amount of Healaflow along the limbus,it is filled in a cannula of desired size. The cannula is then transferred to NaHa syringe and used. The end point is difficult to make out since NaHa and Healaflow are both transparent. The other way is to attach Healaflow carrying cannula to a trypan blue syringe. The moment blue dye is seen, it means that whole of "cannula contained" Healaflow has been delivered. If more Healaflow is desired, the amount can be delivered direct from Healaflow syringe.

Microtrack Filtration plus Healaflow films are here:

Healaflow only:

http://www.youtube.com/watch?v=2wKcwOYdKfc

Healaflow and trypan blue:

http://www.youtube.com/watch?v=CBnJl2riAso

Failed MTF Ologen case, Re-MTF along with Healaflowhttp://www.youtube.com/watch?v=WTWSK1O1c8g

5. Spongy resistance

Collagen matrix (available as Ologen) is a sponge like structure having wide bore channels ranging from 20 to 200 microns.It is available as discs of various sizes and shape, the sizes being 6 to 10 mm and the height being 1 to 2 mm. They have been made with a view to cater for the needs of filtration surgery techniques in which scleral flaps are made. The matrix is said to guide the fibroblasts through the pores in a random fashion and thus prevent scar formation.It may also act as a reservoir buffer to prevent shallow or flat anterior chamber. When wetted it swells up like a sponge. Ologen is said to disappear in 3 months time.

Ologen appears an interesting material to increase subconjunctival resistance to the free flow of aqueous, after MTF. I have used it two ways:

1. Placing a small piece of Ologen in the immediate vicinity or directly over the MTF external pore.

2. Placing multiple Ologen pieces some distance from MTF track, with a view to create resistance to the passage of aqueous, in to the lymphatics.. The swollen Ologen pieces compress the lymphatics in the area.

The steps of operation are as follows:

Anesthesia as usual

1. Make a 0.75 mm pocket incision close to the limbus. Use carbachol intraocular to contract the pupil.

2. Fugo blade iridotomy/iridotomies,as described earlier, followed by irrigation of the anterior chamber to clear the released pigment.

3. Make a hole in the conjunctiva close to the limbus at 10 O'clock. Through this hole a long 30 gauge cannula is introduced under the conjunctiva and is used to loosen the subconjunctiva close to the limbus.

4. A small elongated piece of Ologen is brought close to the conjunctival opening.It swells up immediately by the local moisture.The material is spongy and pliable. It can be pushed under the conjunctiva by the tip of a thin cannula.The Ologen piece is taken to 12 O' clock site close to the limbus. It shrinks when the conjunctiva is pressed, and swells up again when the pressure is released.The Ologen piece may be stained with trypan blue before insertion, for better visualization during the entire process.

5. A 100 micron Fugo blade glaucoma tip is entered with momentary low energy under the conjunctiva about 7-8 mm from the limbus, in line with the Ologen piece. The tip is then pushed unactivated under the conjunctiva and under the Ologen piece, till it reaches real close to the conjunctival attachment to the limbus. The tip is rested there and is then raised to an angle of 30 degree or over, depending upon of the resistance of the conjunctiva, under which it is working.

6. With hand steadily holding the Fugo blade and the tip putting very slight pressure at the limbus, it is momentarily activated from foot switch. It instantly passes through the limbus in to the anterior chamber,as indicated by the formation of cavitation bubbles in the anterior chamber.During passage through the limbus, cavitation bubbles also spread on both sides of the entry point, which makes the corneal tissue temporarily opaque.

7. Air is injected in the anterior chamber.

8. A balloon of 0.1 to 0.2 ml of Mitomycin 0.01 or 0.02 % is made under the conjunctiva.

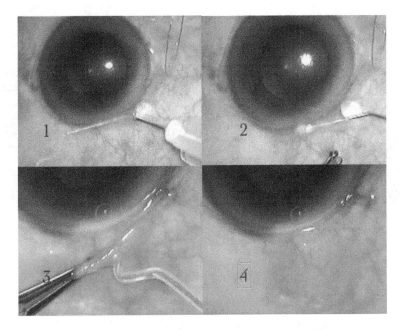

Figure 17. A thin cannula loosens the subconjunctival space close to the limbus.A piece of Ologen is pushed through the conjunctival opening to the 12 O clock limbus.MTF is performed close to one end of Ologen. Air bubble in the anterior chamber is an indication that MTF track really got made.

Postoperatively, we watch the state of the anterior chamber and the bleb and remain awake to the possibility of internal blockage of the track with the iris, the only problem point of MTF surgery.

We have observed that if there is no free movement of aqueous, the collagen matrix becomes hard and dry and refuses to get absorbed.It also becomes adherent to the overlying conjunctiva and it becomes difficult to separate the two.

Healaflow and Ologen are two materials, which can increase the subconjunctival lymphatic resistance to the out coming aqueous. This resistance is important in the first few postoperative weeks. It reduces the chances of shallowing/absence of the anterior chamber. Both materials provide resistance, one as a liquid cushion and the other as a soft sponge. The placement of Healaflow is easier than Ologen. Both materials are supposed to disappear with passage of time. It is not easy to find out when the material disappeared or whether it really disappeared. However our main concern is to see if they did the work that was expected from them i.e. reducing the incidence and severity of internal blockage of the track with iris. After doing 75-80 surgeries in both groups, it is our perception that there has been a palpable reduction in the use of YAG laser for removing internal MTF iris blocks.

There is only one variation possible with Healaflow, namely the amount of the material deposited. With Ologen many variations are possible, namely number, size and position of the pieces.Furthermore, if an Ologen piece is placed at the limbus, MTF track can be made on one side,under it or through it.

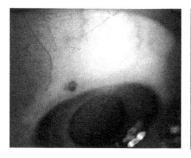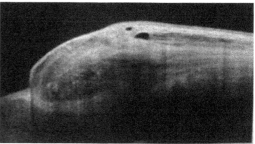

Figure 18. MTF and Ologen, 6 months postoperative. Ologen has caught the pigment coming from inside, that would otherwise have been drained away with aqueous.OCT shows good cover for bleb.It is difficult to decide if Ologen has been absorbed or not.

Here is a film on MTF with Ologen piece over the filtration track:

http://www.youtube.com/watch?v=NkwuIRjA3aQ

To treat hypotony after MTF surgery,we have also used/placed a piece of Ologen directly on the over-filtering MTF track, with success.

6. Reducing the width of the filtration track

The standard 100 micron glaucoma tip has a teflon sleeve of 50 microns thickness.For it to pass through the limbus, the plasma on the tip has to be wider than combined width of the fibre and sleeve. At medium power, the plasma cloud is 50 microns, therefore the track width is 200 microns. At high power setting the plasma cloud is 75 microns on all sides of the filament, therefore the track size is 250 microns. If we use naked filaments of 75, 100 or 120 microns at low energy, we can have smaller widths of MTF tracks. Thinner tracks cause slow decompression during surgery. Since the speed of aqueous out flow gets reduced, the track is less likely to attract the iris.If a block occurs, the iris tissue is small and is easy to dislodge. Some successful cases show no bleb at all.

The steps of mini-MTF operation are as follows:

1. Pocket incision 0.75 mm parallel to the upper limbus.Inject carbachol to contract the pupil.

2. Make a conjunctival opening near 10 O'clock limbus and inject 0.01 or 0.02 % MMC to balloon the conjunctiva along the limbus and beyond.

3. Peripheral iridotomies are done with Fugo blade. The important thing is to wash out completely all the pigment/debris produced during iridotomy, because even a small particle can block the filtration track from inside.

4. Fill the upper part of anterior chamber with NaHa.

5. Push away any subconjunctival fluid close to the limbus, by sweeping with a cannula.

6. For MTF, use a 75 micron naked filament Fugo blade tip.Push the conjunctiva towards the cornea, with a blunt sapphire knife. When the limbal area is clearly seen, the activated tip is passed through the conjunctiva and the limbus in to the anterior chamber. The aqueous does not come out, but the track making is complete,since cavitation bubbles are seen to arise in the anterior chamber. One can make two or more tracks if so desired. A second track can not be made if aqueous has started flowing out, because the naked tip does not work in the water. NaHa in the anterior chamber helps make more than one track.

7. Healaflow may be deposited under the conjunctiva if so desired, at this stage.

8. A small air bubble is placed in the anterior chamber. It pushes out some NaHa and aqueous, proving that the system is working.

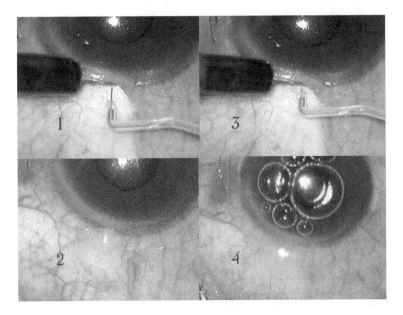

Figure 19. A naked 75 micron Fugo blade tip kept close to the conjunctiva retracting sapphire blunt blade, passes through the conjunctiva and limbus as soon as it is activated.The bleb forms slowly. Air is injected in the anterior chamber at the end.

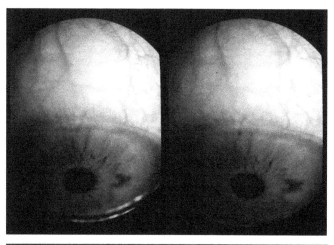

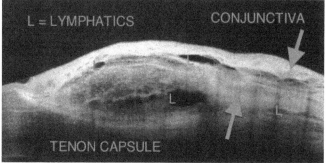

Figure 20. The bleb after Mini-MTF. The anterior chamber has remained well formed.The bleb appearance is reassuring. L are for lymphatics.

Here is a film on small track MTF

http://www.youtube.com/watch?v=WEn_AS_h9Do

7. Mitomycin

MMC reduces scar formation. This helps to improve results. Unlike other surgical techniques in which MMC is applied under the conjunctiva with sponges, we raise a bleb with 0.1 to 0.2 ml of a desired concentration of MMC. This assures a wider spread that results in a borderless bleb.Our OCT observations of the blebs show that MTF cases maintain a healthy cover of the conjunctiva. There is no danger of bleb leakage, because no conjunctival flap is made. MMC concentration has been used varying from 0.005 % to 0.04 %. The higher risk cases receive higher concentration of MMC. The deposited MMC is left as such,its dilution starts as soon as the track is made and aqueous starts draining. The mainstream glaucoma surgery does not give a thought to lymphatics. We believe that they are the crux of successful filtration surgery. It is a great satisfaction that they are not damaged by MMC with the concentration used. An MTF opening is small compared to tracks made with other techniques. Therefore it is all the more important that it should not get scarred on the outside.

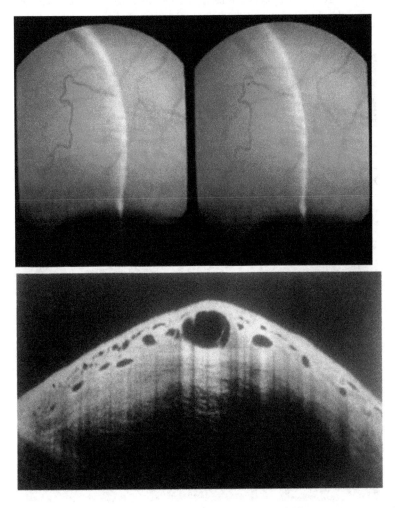

Figure 21. A 35 years old case of MTF, shows the presence of filled lymphatics under the conjunctiva, one month after surgery, both on slit lamp optical section and with OCT. The OCT image is particularly striking. IOP is 9 mm, down from 35 mm.

8. A bandage contact lens

A bandage lens provides a soft lid over the external opening of MTF. It helps to maintain the depth of the anterior chamber. At the time of surgery there is already formed a bleb that prevents it from occupying its intended place. However, after 3-4 hours, when the taped eye is opened, the bandage lens shall be found sitting over the track. The bandage lens may be removed after a week or two. If no bleb is seen under the bandage lens, it is a sign that somehow the iris has blocked the track from inside.

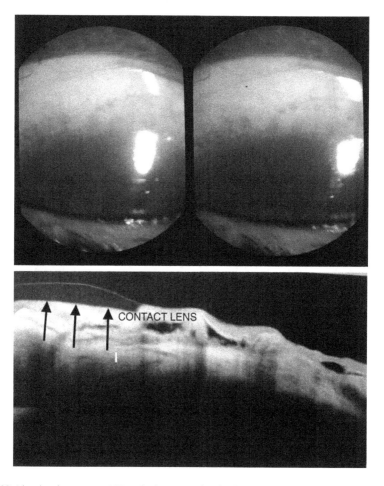

Figure 22. A bandage lens over two MTF tracks. The anterior chamber has good depth. OCT shows a bandage contact lens riding over track area

9. Comments

From the foregoing description many points are clear. MTF is the least traumatic of all filtration operations. Currently we are making 150 to 250 micron filtration tracks. We are trying to cope with the frequent problem of internal block by iris, which has to be cleared with YAG laser. YAG laser management of iris block is a minor intervention.But think of the worldwide lack of YAG lasers in clinics and far off places. All the various strategies described above are attempts to keep the iris away. At the same time filtration should continue. I do all my filtration surgery with a 6X head-worn loupe/microscope. Thus it is possible to perform MTF in any remote area, where the light source shall be a hand held bright LED flash light.No dissection filtration surgery protects conjunctival lymphatics.There is an ever increasing load of tens of millions of glaucoma patients, who can not afford life long medication.

Now let us consider, minimally traumatic filtration surgery in some specific situations.

10. Failed trabeculectomy

The following is a description of a forty years old male who had a failed trabeculectomy surgery.IOP was 41 mm. under multiple medications. The

scleral flap was clearly visible and there was no trace of a bleb.The surgery was done as under:

The conjunctiva was raised with MMC 0.01%. A 100 micron microtrack was made close to the failed area followed by air injection in the anterior chamber.A 300 micron Fugo blade was then used to make a conjunctival opening 7-8 mm proximal to the upper edge of the closed scleral flap.The tip was pushed to the edge of the scleral flap.The tip was activated and insinuated under the edge of closed scleral flap at many places.The subscleral space communication with the anterior chamber was assured. 4 months postoperative, the IOP was 12 mm and the bleb was good.

The movie of this patient is here:

http://youtu.be/T72kVgNeKzY

There are more movies on this topic:

http://www.youtube.com/watch?v=HxZravthPGI

http://www.youtube.com/watch?v=jn7ojuYbmaE

Management of Tenon cyst formation after TCFTCF:

http://www.youtube.com/watch?v=Bo3crwrpUDg

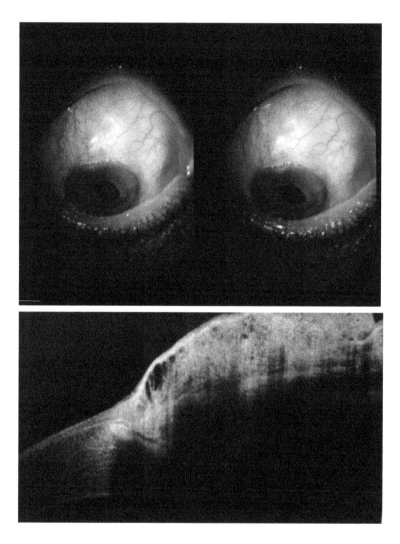

Figure 23. Failed trabeculectomy case, 4 months after MTF and opening the scleral flap with Fugo blade. OCT shows that the bleb is well made and safe.

10.1. Neovascular glaucoma

TCTCF is the least traumatic way of filtration surgery in neovascular glaucoma.The track avoids the new vessel formation in the iris and angle.Decompression may start bleeding in the angle, but it does not affect the filtration through TCF track.

A film on TCTCF in an already failed glaucoma surgery is seen here:

http://www.youtube.com/watch?v=uO57F9gdTU4

10.2. Buphthalmos

Buphthalmos is one of the most difficult conditions to treat. Failures are common. Therefore it is important that any glaucoma surgery should not leave behind a large foot print on the sclera and the overlying tissues. With the standard approaches, we run short of surgical space and options very soon. Then comes the turn of destructive procedures. Our technique of choice is MTF with or without additional measures to improve chances of success.TCTCF is less commonly employed. The surgery might succeed on the very first attempt or after many attempts. There always remains a chance of successfully doing another atraumatic filtration operation.

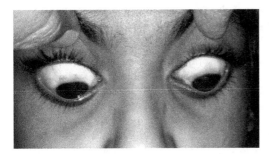 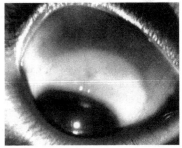

Figure 24. A ten year old buphthalmos child who had MTF 5 years before. The surgery was successful on the very first attempt. In both eyes IOP is 12 mm without medication.MMC 0.01 was used to balloon the conjunctiva at the beginning of surgery. There was a wait period of 4 minutes, before MTF was done.

A few films on MTF in buphthalmos are here:

MTF for buphthalmos, Healaflow put under the conjunctiva at the end:

http://www.youtube.com/watch?v=glddXJmSOeg

TCTCF in a case of pediatric glaucoma (patient 10 years old).Mitomycin injected under the conjunctiva at the end:

http://www.youtube.com/watch?v=Xfe6ac659Xc

Another MTF for buphthalmos:

http://www.youtube.com/watch?v=ezIJ_8HIeMM

Micro-spherophakia and buphthalmos:

http://www.youtube.com/watch?v=yM-raYTKdcg&feature=relmfu

10.3. Pseudophakic pupil block glaucoma

Through one or more 0.7 mm pocket incisions in the cornea, Fugo blade 100 micron glaucoma tip is introduced and many iridotomies are done to completely overcome the pupillary block. This may be followed by MTF or TCTCF.

A few films on the topic are seen here:

http://www.youtube.com/watch?v=etyBCd4pWoU

http://www.youtube.com/watch?v=CtgNZGwFOJU

http://www.youtube.com/watch?v=8R_n729PWno

11. Concluding remarks

An estimated 80 million (and increasing by millions every year) cases of glaucoma patients worldwide are a challenge to the ingenuity of the surgeons and the producers of glaucoma medications and devices.

We have understood the presence and importance of lymphatics under the conjunctiva and in the adjoining tissues. We have tried to preserve the lymphatics by minimally invasive techniques of TCTCF and especially MTF. Besides new surgical innovations, we have also made use of newer viscoelastic and spongy materials in the hope of preserving the filtration tracks as well as saving the conjunctival lymphatics. Much work/research remains to be done before we and other workers in the field can declare a victory over the worldwide blinding epidemic of glaucoma. Needless to say, Fugo blade is helpful in making TCF and MTF tracks. As yet there is no other tool that can do the same.

Author details

Daljit Singh

Guru Nanak Dev University, Amritsar, India

References

[1] Bethke WC. A New Clue to Lymphatic Drainage? Review of Ophthalmology. 2002; 9, 3

[2] Dow T, Devenecia G. Transciliary Filtration (Singh Filtration) with the Fugo Plasma Blade. Ann Ophthalmol. 2008; 40,1; 8-14

[3] Eisenstein P. World's Smallest Knives. Popular Mechanics. 2003; 180, 10; 56-8.

[4]   Fine IH, Hoffman RS, Packer M. Highlights of the 2002 ASCRS Symposium, Part I. Eyeworld. 2002;7,7:38

[5]   Fugo R. Regarding Transciliary Filtration. Tropical Ophthalmology. 2002; 2, 1; 7-8.

[6]   Fugo R. Transciliary Filtration Procedure Offers New Approach to Glaucoma. Ocular Surg News. 2005; 16,6; 18-19.

[7]   Fugo RJ. Trans-ciliary Filtration. Video Journal of Current Glaucoma Practices. Sept-Dec. 2007. Vol. 1, No. 2.

[8]   Fugo RJ. Plasma blade has several applications in ophthalmic surgery. Ocular Surg News. Dec 25, 2009

[9]   Guttman C. Anterior segment tool proves ideal for many applications. Ophthalmology Times. 2005;30,2;14,16.

[10] Guttman C. Transciliary filtration provides improved safety and simplicity. Ophthalmology Times. 2005;30,3; 28.

[11] Izak AM, Werner L, Pandey SK, Apple DJ, Izak MGJ. Analysis of the capsule edge after Fugo plasma blade capsulotomy, continuous curvilinear capsulorhexis, and can-opener capsulotomy. J Cataract Refract Surg. 2004;30, 12;2606-2611.

[12] Kent C. Revealed: the Eye's Lymphatic System. Ophthalmic Manage. 2002; 6, 5: 114.

[13] McGrath, D. Fugo Blade effective tool for multiple surgical applications. Eurotimes. 2008; 13, 6:43.

[14] Peponis V, Rosenberg P, Reddy SV, Herz JB, Kaufman HE. The Use of the Fugo Blade in Corneal Surgery: A preliminary Animal Study. Cornea. 2006; 2: 206-8.

[15] Pollack,I.P.(2000).Ocular Surgery News.Europe/Asia Pacific Edition,July 1,2000.

[16] Ronge L. How to Use the Fugo Blade. EyeNet. 2003; 7, 9; 23-4.

[17] Roy,H.,Singh,D.,Fugo.R.Ocular Applications of Fugo Blade.(2010) Lippincots Williams and Wilkins,p.77 -126.

[18] (Roy,S,Thi HD,Feusier M and Mermoud A (2012).Crosslinked sodium hyaluronate implant in deep sclerectomy for the surgical treatment of glaucoma. European Journal of ophthalmology,Vol 22,No.2.pp 70-76 (2012).

[19] Scimeca G. Phaco with Transciliary Filtration an Alternative to Triple Procedure. Ocular Surg News. 2005; 23,11; 58.

[20] Singh D. Singh Micro-Filtration for Glaucoma; A New Technique. Tropical Ophthalmology. 2001; 1, 6: 7-11.

[21] Singh D, Singh K. Transciliary Filtration Using the Fugo Blade. Ann Ophthalmol. 2002; 34,3; 183-87

[22] Singh D. Letters: Conjunctival Lymphatic System. J Cataract Refract Surg. 2003; 29, 4; 632-3.

[23] Singh D. Transciliary Filtration & Lymphatics of Conjunctiva- A Tale of Discovery. Tropical Ophthalmology. 2002; 2, 1; 9-13

[24] Singh D, Singh RSJ, Singh K, Singh SK, Singh IR, Singh R, Fugo RJ. The Conjunctival Lymphatic System. Ann Ophthalmol. 2003;35, 2;99-

[25] Singh D.Microtrack Filtration. Annals of Ophthalmology 2002;34,3;183-187

[26] Trivedi RH, Wilson Jr. ME, Bartholomew LR. Extensibility and scanning electron microscopy evaluation of 5 pediatric anterior capsulotomy techniques in a porcine model. J Cataract Refract Surg. 2006; 32, 7:1206-13.

[27] Winn CW. Broad applications seen for electrosurgical instrument. Ocular Surg News. 2001; 19, 11: 45-46

[28] Yeni H et al. Identification of lymphatics in the ciliary body of the human eye: A novel "uveolymphatic" outflow pathway.Experimental Eye Research 89 (2009) 810–819

Chapter 8

Combined Cataract-Glaucoma Surgery

Vassilis Kozobolis,
Aristeidis Konstantinidis and
Georgios Labiris

Additional information is available at the end of the chapter

1. Introduction

Glaucoma is an optic neuropathy which causes a characteristic loss of optic nerve fibers. The loss of the nerve fibers leads to an increase of the optic disc cupping with subsequent visual field defects [1]. It is estimated that around 60 million people suffer from open angle and closed angle glaucoma with the majority of the patients being female and 47% living in Asia. Another 6 million people suffer from various forms of secondary glaucoma. The patients blind from glaucoma are around 8 million [2,3]. The glaucoma is the second cause of blindness worldwide following cataract.

The aim of the treatment of the glaucoma is the lowering of the intraocular pressure (IOP) as research shown that the higher the IOP the higher the risk of developing glaucoma [4]. In the developed countries the first treatment option is the use of IOP lowering drops while in the developing world trabeculectomy is the first option. Trabeculectomy was regarded as an excellent option for the initial management of glaucoma before the introduction of the newer antiglaucoma drops [6]. Later research showed that patients on topical medication had better quality of life compared to those who underwent trabeculectomy although trabeculectomy was more efficient in lowering the IOP [7]. The introduction of newer and more potent drops as well as further research that showed the failure of trabeculectomy over time, limited the initial enthusiasm of the surgical approach as the initial management of glaucoma [8,9]. This led to a decrease in the number of trabeculectomies performed every year in the developed countries from mid 1990's [10-14].

2. Glaucoma surgery overview

Surgical techniques of the glaucoma surgery include:

- the penetrating techniques (trabeculectomy and its variations)
- the non-penetrating techniques (deep sclerectomy, viscocanalostomy, canaloplasty)
- the glaucoma drainage devices
  - with valve (Ahmed, Krupin)
  - without valve (Molteno, Baerveldt)
  - mini shunt (Ex-PRESS)
- newer devices (Glaukos iStent, Eyepass, Trabektome, CyPass, Solx gold shunt, Aquashunt, endophotocoagulation)
- The trabecular aspiration in pseudoexfoliation glaucoma

The concept of minimally invasive glaucoma surgery (MIGS) has gained a lot of interest in the recent years. The aim of these procedures is to minimize the side affects of the classic trabeculectomy by avoiding the formation of a large filtering bleb. The primary indication for MIGS is early to moderate open-angle glaucoma as they tend not to lower the IOP as much as trabeculectomy. The classification of MIGS can vary according to the surgical technique used, the formation of a filtering bleb and the aqueous dynamics

2.1. Classification of MIGS

Surgical technique

- **Ab interno** (Glaukos iStent, Trabektome, Cypass, Eyepass, Aquashunt, Solx Gold microshunt)
- **Ab externo** (canaloplasty)

Bleb formation

- **Bleb related** (Deep sclerectomy)
- **Blebless** (canaloplasty, Glaukos iStent, Trabektome, CyPass, Eyepass, Aquashunt, Solx Gold microshunt)

Aqueous dynamics

- Increasing outflow through the trabeculum (canaloplasty)
- Increasing outflow through collector channels (trabectome, Glaukos iStent, Eyepass)
- Increasing outflow through suprachoroidal space (CyPass, Solx Gold microshunt, Aquashunt)

All the above techniques can be combined with simultaneous cataract extraction.

3. Combined cataract–glaucoma surgery

Indications

The main indications for combined surgery are:

- the presence of cataract and medically uncontrolled glaucoma

- advanced glaucoma and cataract which is likely to progress soon after an antiglaucoma surgical procedure

- the early treatment of glaucoma in cataract patients

Pros

- Decreased risk of one surgical and anaesthetic procedure compared to two different procedures

- Less cost to healthcare services

- Less operating time

- Faster visual rehabilitation

- Decreased incidence of postoperative pressure spikes compared to cataract surgery alone

Cons

- Lengthy procedure that requires experience

- A complicated cataract surgery may compromise the success of the antiglaucoma procedure

The procedure that the surgeon will undertake first largely depends on the level of the IOP and the severity of the glaucomatous damage. It is known that phacoemulsification has a small hypotensive effect [15,16, 17]. Phacoemulsification can be considered first when the there is mild glaucomatous damage which progresses very slowly (as assessed by fundoscopy and standard automated perimetry), the IOP is in the mid twenties and the patient's main concern is poor vision due to cataract. Furthermore cataract extraction can take place first if there is a bulky cataractous crystalline lens that is the most likely cause of an elevated IOP.

Trabeculectomy should be considered first if the glaucomatous damage is extensive and/or the IOP is very high and when the cataract operation is likely to intervene with the success of the glaucoma filtering procedure (e.g.: zonular instability due to pseudoexfoliation). The surgeon should be aware of the fact that phacoemulsification following trabeculectomy has a adverse effect on the survival of the antiglaucoma procedure [18]

The combined procedure should be considered when there is significant cataract in the presence of significant glaucomatous damage in a patient whose cataract operation is likely to be uneventful or when the patient would not like to have two separate procedures done or the surgeon feels that it is risky for a particular patient to be taken to theatre twice.

3.1. Anaesthetic considerations

The combined surgery can be done under general anaesthesia, retro/peribulbar or sub-Tenon's block or with topical anaesthesia. All topical blocks are carried out with the patient lying on the operating bed. We use a mixture of 1:1 lidocaine 2% and bupivacaine 0.5%.

We perform retrobulbar anaesthesia with a 23G needle. The inferior orbital rim is palpated through the skin at the junction of its middle and lateral thirds and the needle is inserted through the skin just above the rim with the patient looking straight ahead. It is then advanced parallel to the orbital floor and when the 4/5 of the length of the needle have been advanced it is slightly retracted and then redirected upwards and slightly nasally to enter the muscle cone. The plunge is retracted to check for blood reflux (blood reflux indicates that the needle may have entered a vessel and the mixture may be injected in the blood circulation). Five to 7 ml of the mixture are injected. Immediate drooping of the upper eyelid is an indication that the anaesthetic is being injected in the muscle cone. Retro/peribulbar block offers excellent anaesthesia and akinesia. The main complications are: globe perforation, retrobulbar haemorrhage, central retinal artery occlusion (due to severe and untreated retrobulbar haemorrhage), and inadvertent brain stem brainstem anaesthesia due to puncture of the meningeal sheaths of the optic nerve and injection of the anaesthetic agents in the cerebrospinal fluid circulation. As the risk of globe rupture increases with the axial length of the eye it should be avoided in big eyes as well as in patients who receive anticoagulants.

The subtenon's block is done as follows: after topical anaesthesia with tetracaine drops, a speculum is inserted and the conjunctiva and Tenon's capsule are grasped with serrated forceps 5-7 mm from the limbus in the inferonasal or inferotemporal quadrant. A fold of conjunctiva is raised with the forceps and a small incision is made with Westcott scissors. A subtenon's canula is inserted through the incision and in closed contact with the globe it is advanced around and behind the eye. Three to 5 ml of the anaesthetic mixture are injected. If the canula is in the subtenon's space then there should not be any conjunctival chemosis. Presence of significant chemosis indicates that the canula lies in the subconjunctival rather than the subtenon's space. The surgeon should make a deeper incision through both conjunctiva and Tenon's capsule and guide the canula behind the globe in close contact with the globe. Subtenon's block also offers adequate anaesthesia but less good akinesia. The most common complications are: subconjunctival haemorrhage and conjunctival chemosis. The risk of globe perforation is minimized as the subtenon's canula is blunt.

Topical anaesthesia is provided with tetracaine drops and Visthesia ampoules containing 2% lidocaine. It is the least invasive procedure but it does not offer akinesia. As the iris is not anaesthetized the patient may be more uncomfortable during the operation compared to the above techniques especially during the iridectomy.

General anaesthesia is seldom done and it is more suitable for claustrophobic patients or those who cannot lie flat and still for lengthy periods of time. In the case of general anaesthesia, retro/ peribulbal and subtenon's block the eye needs to be rotated downwards with the use of a traction suture (described later) in order to expose the superior bulbar conjunctiva.

4. Combined phacoemulsification–trabeculectomy

4.1. One–site versus two–site combined surgery

There is evidence that the two-site surgery offers slightly lower IOP (1-3 mmHg) than the one-site surgery [19-21]. The authors favor the two-site technique as it causes less damage to the area of filtration and subsequently less fibrosis with better chances for the survival of the trabeculectomy over time.

In the one-site technique the main incision of the phacoemulsification is done under the sclera flap and the corneoscleral block excision is done at the site of the main incision. In the two-site approach the main incision of the phacoemulsification is done 90° away from the trabeculectomy site and towards the temporal side of the eye.

In the surgeons' experience there was no significant difference in the IOP control between the two approaches.

4.2. Limbus versus fornix conjunctival incision

The limbus and fornix based conjunctival flaps are equally effective in lowering IOP [22-24]. However there is evidence that limbus based flaps are more prone to late hypotony and bleb infection [22,25]. Early bleb leaks were more common in the fornix based flaps [23,24].

4.3. Aqueous humor dynamics in trabeculectomy

The aim of the trabeculectomy is to bypass the conventional outflow pathway through the trabeculum and Schlemm's canal. The aqueous humor flows through an internal ostium at the level of the trabeculum under the scleral flap in the subconjunctiva/sub-Tenon's space with the formation of a filtering bleb. The scleral flap reduces the unrestricted flow of aqueous and can be secured to the sclera with fixed, releasable or adjustable sutures. A peripheral iridectomy at the site of the operation prevents the peripheral iris from obstructing the internal ostium. In some cases such as pseudophakic or myopic eyes where the peripheral iris rests well away from the ostium the peripheral iridectomy can be avoided. In this way the chances of hyphaema and significant postoperative inflammation are reduced.

4.4. Risk factors in trabeculectomy

The long term success of the trabeculectomy depends on several risk factors:

- *Black race*. The AGIS study showed weak evidence that Afro-Caribbean origin is a risk factor for failed trabeculectomy [26]. The results by Scott et al [27] agree with AGIS outcomes. However two studies by Sturmer et al [28] and Broadway et al [29] did not show statistically significant differences. The latter publication although it reports higher success rate in white patients it concludes that this difference was not statistically different. The authors speculate that trabeculectomy generally is considered to be less successful in black patients and the reason for that being their younger age during surgery and the fact that Tenon's capsule is capable of producing more intense inflammatory and subsequently fibrotic response.

- *Young age*. There is conflicting evidence in the literature as to whether young age is a risk factor for failed trabeculectomy. While the AGIS study [26] and Broadway et al [29] report that trabeculectomy has less favourable outcome overtime in young patients, other studies do not confirm these findings [28,30]

- *Combined procedure*. Research shows that combined phacotrabeculectomy produces lower hypotensive effect than trabeculectomy alone (discussed later)

- *Long term treatment with multiple antiglaucoma drops*. There is strong evidence that long term treatment with antiglaucoma drops increases the number of inflammatory cells [31] and decreases the success of trabeculectomy [32]

- *Previous operations*. Subconjunctival scarring from previous operations can limit the success of the trabeculectomy. The AGIS study [26] did not identify repeat trabeculectomies (second or third trabeculectomy) as a risk factor for failure. A possible explanation may be that repeat trabeculectomies were done with the use of antifibrotic agents. Indeed Broadway et al [33] reported that trabeculectomies following conjunctival incisional operations were more likely to fail compared to primary trabeculectomies More recent studies confirmed that repeat trabeculectomies augmented by intraoperative use of mitonycin C is an effective procedure for IOP control [34,35]

- *Secondary glaucomas (traumatic, uveitic, aphakic, rubeotic)*. Mietz et al [36] found that the neovascular, traumatic and uveitic glaucoma had the worst prognosis regarding trabeculectomy survival.

- *Diabetes*. The AGIS study as well as a study by Hugkulstone et al [37] found that diabetes is a risk factor for failed trabeculectomy

4.5. Antifibrotic agents

4.5.1. Antimetabolites

Despite the initial success of the trabeculectomy clinical experience has shown that the operation tends to fail over time. This is due to the postoperative inflammation and the resulting formation of scar tissue at the site of the operation especially in the subconjunctival space. In order to improve the success of the operation surgeons resort to the use of antimetabolites namely mitomycin C (MMC) and 5-fluorouracil (5-FU) [38]. They both inhibit fibroblast proliferation: 5-FU is antagonizes pyrimidine activity and inhibits DNA synthesis and thus suppresses fibroblast activity and inhibits epithelial cell proliferation while mitomycin C which is an alkylating agent interferes with all phases of cell cycle and prevents fibroblast and endothelial cell replication. MMC is more potent and has a more lasting in vivo effect than 5-FU. They can be used both intraoperatively and postoperatively. When used during surgery MMC was found to be slightly more effective than 5-FU with comparable rate of side effects [39]. The intraoperative dose of 5-FU is 0.1 ml of a 50mg/ml solution for 5 minutes. MMC has been used in varying concentration (0.2-0.4mg/ml) and application time (2-5 minutes) depending on the severity of glaucoma and presence of risk factors. The authors prefer the use of lasik shields soaked in the antimetabolite solution under the conjunctiva and after the formation of the scleral flap.

Evidence has shown that the use of antimetabolites during surgery is associated with better IOP control [40,41]. On the other hand the use of antimetabolites has increased the incidence of side effects such as the postoperative hypotony, toxicity of the corneal epithelium, early and delayed bleb leaks, blebitis and endophthalmitis [42-44]. The antimetabolites can also be used postoperatively with bleb needling in cases of failing blebs.

4.5.2. Corticosteroids and non–steroidal anti–inflammatory drugs (NSAIDs)

It is well established that the postoperative use of topical steroids is associated with better IOP control and less glaucoma medicines [45]. Corticosteroids can be used in a preemptive fashion before surgery in patients who were treated with antiglaucoma drops as these patients have lower success rate [46,47]. Research has shown that the instillation of corticosteroids and NSAIDs before surgery leads to better outcomes in terms of likelihood of bleb needling and postoperative use of antiglaucoma drops [48]. The injection of triamcinolone in the bleb or behind the globe seems beneficial in terms of IOP control [49-51]

4.5.3. Anti–VEGF

Recently bevacizumab has been used intraoperatively instead of MMC in order to improve the success rate of the trabeculectomy but it has not proved to be superior to MMC [52,53].

4.6. Pre–operative preparation

The authors do not routinely prescribe topical corticosteroids before the antiglaucoma procedures unless the conjunctiva is markedly inflamed. In this case fluorometholone drops are given four times per day for one month before the operation. If the IOP is unacceptably high and there is high risk of expulsive haemorrhage tablets acetozolamide 250 mg 4 times per day are given for one or two days preoperatively. Additionally 200-400 ml of intravenous mannitol 20% are administered over 45-60 minutes on the morning before the operation. In theatre the eye is first anaesthetized with topical medication and then the local block is given according to the surgeon's preference. The skin around the eye is cleaned with iodine povidone solution 10%. A sterile drape is placed over the eye and a diluted 5% iodine solution is instilled on the eye and conjunctival fornices to achieve asepsis of the ocular surface.

4.7. Surgical technique

The following steps are the technique of choice of the authors for the combined phacoemulsi-fication-trabeculectomy procedure:

- 7/0 Vicryl corneal traction suture 4 mm from the limbus (optional)

- Blunt conjunctival and Tenon's dissection over a wide area. We try to limit limbal peritomy to three o' clock hours in order to achieve watertight closure with as few sutures as possible. Dissection is carried out posteriorly towards the insertion of the superior rectus muscle

- Scleral flap formation (4×4mm) at 50% of the sclera thickness. Initially we perform a sclera incision 4mm long 4mm behind the limbus. Scleral dissection is performed with a beveled crescent knife until the limbal vessels are reached. Then we perform the side cuts to create the sclera flap.

- Application of MMC (0.2 mg/ml for 2-3 minutes) with the use of a few pieces of of a lasik shield arranged over a wide area under the conjunctiva. The edges of the conjunctiva are grasped with serrated forceps and are wiped with Weck-cell sponges in order to remove MMC. The presence of MMC at the cut edge of the conjunctiva may prevent wound closure and lead to postoperative leak.

- The area of application of MMC is then irrigated with 20 ml of balanced salt solution

- Bipolar cautery is kept to a minimum

- 2.75 mm clear cornea phacoemulsification from a temporal approach with injectable intraocular lens insertion

- Balanced salt solution (BSS) injection in the stroma or a 10/0 nylon suture at the site of the main incision of the phacoemulsification in order to encourage filtration though the scleral flap rather than the main incision. As BSS induced stromal oedema lasts for a very short period of time we prefer to close the main incision with a suture

- Pre-placement of two 10/0 Nylon releasable sutures at the two corners of the flap (fig 1). We prefer to pre-place the sutures in order to reduce the period of hypotony during the creation of the internal ostium and peripheral iridectomy

- Entry in the anterior chamber at the site of the scleral flap

- Excision of a corneoscleral block (internal ostium) with a Kelly punch.

- Peripheral iridectomy (if needed). This step can be omitted in cases of highly myopic and pseudophakic in which case the iris lies quite posteriorly from the internal ostium

- Tying of the scleral flap releasable sutures (more sutures can be used according to the surgeon's discretion). This step is very critical as the surgeon checks the amount of aqueous flowing from the edges of the sclera flap. Ideally there should be some "oozing" only, after BSS is slowly injected from side ports of the phacoemulsification

- Conjunctival and Tenon's layer closure in one plane with 10/0 nylon sutures. Usually two sutures (one at each side of the limbal peritomy) are used and tied in a purse-string fashion. One or two horizontal mattress sutures are used between the first sutures. The conjunctival wound is then checked for leakage.

- Triamcinolone or celectone chronodose injection subconjunctivally 0.1 ml behind the scleral flap at the end of the operation. 0.1 ml of gentamycin (solution of 80 mg in 2ml) is injected subconjunctivally in the lower fornix.

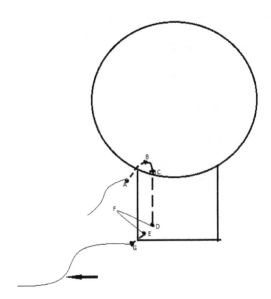

Figure 1. Technique for inserting a releasable suture. A: first entry of suture just behind the limbus, B: first exit of suture into clear cornea just in front of the limbus, C: second entry of suture into clear cornea just in front of the limbus. The suture runs through the thickness of the sclera flap and exits at point D, E:third entry point of suture through the full thickness of the sclera flap and exits at point G in the sclera. The free end of the suture (arrow) is tied with 4 throws to the loop F. The suture is not locked. It can be removed by pulling the small loop between points B and C. It is important that the suture runs at an angle of 45° between points E and G in order to pull the flap both laterally and posteriorly.

4.8. Postoperative management

Cyclopentolate drops 1% are given 3 times per day for 2-3 weeks in order to reduce the intraocular inflammation and reduce the incidence of aqueous misdirection. Drops dexamethasone 0.1% and tobramycin 0.3% 8 times per day are gives in the immediate postoperative period. The frequency is reduced according to the postoperative course of the operation. If the there is anterior chamber or conjunctival inflammation the drops should be given more frequently and for longer periods of time. While the antibiotic drops can be discontinued after 4 weeks, steroids may need to be continued for 6 months at a low frequency (e.g.: 1 drop/day or on alternate days). If there are signs of subconjunctival scarring (dilated vessels that do not run smoothly on the conjunctiva but seem distorted along their course), subconjunctival dexamethasone 0.1 ml (8mg in 2ml solution) and 5FU 0.1 ml (10 ml solution containing 500 mg) injections can be administered not more frequently than weekly injections. The injections are done just behind the bleb. The insertion of the needle should be at least 5mm away from the bleb in order to avoid bleb leakage after the needle is withdrawn.

Needling may be needed if the there is scarring. We perform the needling at the slit lamp as follows: the eye is anaesthetized with tetracaine 1% and Visthesia ampoules. Asepsis of the ocular surface is achieved with 5% iodine povidone solution. A 30G needle mounted on a insulin syringe containing BSS is inserted under the conjunctiva at least 5mm away from the bleb. BSS is slowly injected to lift the conjunctiva and the needle is directed towards the site of the bleb. Subconjunctival fibrosis is broken with sweeping movements of the needle. If the anterior chamber is to be entered a Hoskins lens is used to deturgess the conjunctiva. The tip of the needle is used to cut the fibrous tissue around the edges of the sclera flap and lift the flap. The needle then enters the anterior chamber through the internal ostium. A mixture of 0.1 ml dexamethasone and 0.1 ml 5 FU is injected through the same entering point behind the bleb.

Argon laser suturolysis can be performed when the sclera flap sutures are tight and obstruct aqueous outflow. The settings are 50μ spot size, 150-250 mW power, 0.1 seconds exposure time through a Hoskins lens.

4.9. Outcomes

There is evidence that combined cataract-glaucoma surgery produces slightly lower hypotensive effect than trabeculectomy alone. [54]

4.10. Complications

The complications of the combined cataract-glaucoma surgery include those of phacoemulsification and those of trabeculectomy. In this chapter we analyze the most common complications of trabeculectomy. It should be noted that a complicated cataract surgery can compromise the success of the trabeculectomy mainly due to the presence of intense inflammation, vitreous or blood in the anterior chamber.

Intraoperative:

- Conjunctival buttonhole. Management: suturing with 10/0 nylon

- Hyphaema

   Mechanism: bleeding from the peripheral iridectomy

   Management: none if it is minimal, aspiration of blood if it stains the cornea or the IOP is high ("/>30 mmHg for 5 days or "/>50 mmHg for two days)

Postoperative

The postoperative complications can broadly be divided in early (which occur 6 weeks after surgery) and late (which occur after 6 weeks from surgery)

Early postoperative:

- High IOP with deep anterior chamber

- Retained viscoelestic. Management: observation, antiglaucoma drops. If IOP is very high it can be aspirated in theatre

- Steroid response. Management: antiglaucoma drops, non-steroidal anti-inflammatory drugs

● Resistance at the level of sclerostomy

Causes:

● Blood. Management: topical steroids, ocular massage, intracameral tissue plasminogen activator [55], aspiration in theatre.

● Iris: retraction of iris tissue with argon laser, removal of iris in theatre.

● Vitreous: YAG-laser to release vitreous, removal of vitreous in theatre.

● Resistance at the level of scleral flap

Causes:

● Tight sutures. Management: ocular massage, argon laser suturolysis, removal of releasable sutures

● Blood. Management: topical steroids, ocular massage, intracameral tissue plasminogen activator, aspiration in theatre.

● Resistance at the level of conjunctiva/Tenon's layer

Causes

Diffuse scar tissue formation or formation of encapsulated bleb (Tenon's cyst). Management. Topical steroids, bleb needling with 5-FU or MMC injection, scar tissue removal in theatre.

There are several signs that will help the clinician to identify the site of obstruction. Gonioscopy will reveal the causes of the obstruction at the level of the internal ostium. Resistance at the level of the sclera flap will produce a very low bleb with no intraepithelial cysts (which are a sign of ample aqueous flow). Resistance at the subconjunctival level with diffuse scar formation will produce a low or slightly elevated bleb with microcysts formation at some areas of the bleb. The conjunctival vessels may be dilated (due to inflammation and subsequent scar tissue deposition) and they can appear "kinked" at some points along their course. Tenon's cyst is a high dome shaped, localized and avascular bleb without microcysts. There may be some engorged vessels on its surface. They typically appear 2-6 weeks after surgery.

● High IOP with shallow anterior chamber

Causes

● Pupillary block. Management: YAG laser/surgical iridectomy. The setting that we use for YAG laser iridectmy are: single or double pulsed shots, defocused posteriorly with starting energy at 5 mJoules

● Suprachoroidal haemorrhage. Management: cycloplegia, topical and systemic steroids, evacuation of blood through sclerostomies in the case of kissing choroidals.

● Aqueous misdirection. Management: mydriatics, aqueous suppressants, YAG laser disruption of the anterior vitreous face, vitrectomy (it disrupts the anterior hyaloids)

● Low IOP with deep/shallow anterior chamber

Risk factors: male gender, young age myopia, MMC [56-58]

Causes

● Overfiltration. Management: pressure patch, large diameter contact lens, cryotherapy, suturing of the scleral flap

- Bleb leak. Management: pressure patch, large diameter contact lens, cyanoacrylate glue, autologous blood, suturing of the conjunctiva

- Aqueous shutdown. Management: topical steroids

- Cyclodialysis cleft. Management: mydriatics, laser photocoagulation/cryotherapy/suturing of the cleft with 7/0 or 8/0 nylon sutures as the 10/0 nylon may not be strong enough the hold the cleft closed if the IOP increases dramatically in the early postoperative period.

In the presence of a very shallow anterior chamber management should include reformation of the anterior chamber with viscoelastic and if there are large choroidal effusions which touch each other (kissing choroidals) then they must be drained via sclerostomies. If the choroidal effusions are not touching each other they can be conservatively managed with cycloplegics, topical steroids. Periocular and oral steroids can also be given

Late postoperative

- Late bleb failure

Causes: scarring. Management: bleb needling, injection of 5-FU/MMC, trabeculectomy revision/redo, glaucoma drainage implants

- Late bleb leak

Cause: thin walled bleb. Risk factors: antimetabolites. Management: aqueous suppressants, large diameter bandage contact lens, autologous serum, cyanoacrylic glue, autologous blood injection in the bleb, conjunctival excision with conjunctival advancement or flap

- Blebitis and bleb related endophthalmitis

Causes: infection of the bleb by various micro-organisms.

Risk factors: thin walled blebs, bleb leaks, exposed sutures, antimetabolites, blepharitis, conjunctivitis, nasolacrimal duct obstruction, diabetes.

Management: sample cultures, broad-spectrum antibiotics (for blebitis), vitreous tap, intravitreal antibiotics ± vitrectomy (for bleb related endophthalmitis)

- Persistent hypotony due to MMC effect (toxic effect on the ciliary body) [59,60]

5. Combined phacoemulsification–non penetrating glaucoma surgery (NPGS)[deep sclerectomy (DS)–Viscocanalostomy (VC)]

5.1. Aqueous humor dynamics in NPGS

The search for a filtering surgery that would minimize the complications of the penetrating surgery has led to the development of the non penetrating procedures in which the anterior chamber is not entered. The aqueous from the anterior chamber percolates through the trabeculo-Descemet's membrane (TDM) either in the episcleral space and then in the subconjunctival/sub-Tenon's space (fig 2), or in the Schlemm's canal (SC) and suprachoroidal space. As the aqueous diffuses to routes other that the subconjunctival/sub-Tenon's space these procedures do not always show elevated filtering blebs. This is especially true for viscocanalostomy in which the aqueous is directed in the enlarged SC and the tight suturing of the scleral flap is considered as a crucial part of the surgical procedure.

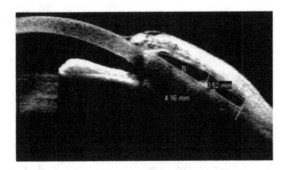

Figure 2. Aqueous in the subconjunctival space flowing DS. A: bleb wall, B: bleb cavity (courtesy of Prof Kozobolis).

5.2. Indications

The main indication for combined phaco-NPGS is the primary open and secondary open angle glaucomas in the presence of visually debilitating cataract.

5.3. Contraindications

Non penetrating glaucoma surgery is useful in open angle glaucomas but should be avoided in closed angle glaucomas as the peripheral iris in these cases blocks the TDM and obstructs the percolation of aqueous. NPGS has also been used in congenital and juvenile glaucomas [61-63].

5.4. Antimetabolites

The adjunctive use of MMC in NPGS showed better hypotensive effect at the cost of higher rate of complications (thin avascular blebs, transconjunctival oozing) [64,65].

5.5. Pre–operative preparation

The same principles apply for the pre-operative preparation as for trabeculectomy

5.6. Surgical technique

The following steps are the technique of choice of the authors for the combined phacoemulsi-fication-DS procedure:

- 7/0 Vicryl corneal traction suture 4 mm from the limbus (optional)

- Conjunctival and Tenon's dissection. As for trabeculectomy we try to keep the limbal peritomy as small as possible

- Application of MMC (0.2 mg/ml for 2-3 minutes) with the use of a few pieces of a lasik shield under the conjunctiva. The edges of the conjunctiva are lifted and wiped off the MMC solution

- The area of MMC application is then irrigated with 20 ml of balanced salt solution

- Bipolar cautery is kept to a minimum

- Formation of a superficial scleral flap at 1/3 of sclera thickness. After the sclera incisions the sclera is dissected anteriorly with a diamond knife until it projects for 1.5 mm into clear cornea

- 2.75 mm clear cornea phacoemulsification from a temporal approach with injectable intraocular lens insertion

- 10/0 nylon suture at the site of the main incision of the phacoemulsification

- The superficial flap is then everted over the cornea and a second deeper triangular scleral flap is dissected under high magnification leaving a very thin layer of scleral tissue over the uvea.

- This second flap is dissected anteriorly in order to deroof Schlemm's canal followed by the removal of the inner wall of SC and the juxtacanalicular trabeculum with the purpose of increasing the aqueous outflow (fig 3)

- Excision of the deep scleral flap

- The superficial scleral flap is repositioned and secured with two 10/0 nylon sutures in a tent – like formation

- Viscoelastic (sodium hyaluronate 1%) is then injected under the scleral flap in order to create a space for the pooling of the aqueous humor

- Conjunctival and Tenon's layer closure in one plane with 10/0 nylon sutures in the same fashion as for trabeculectomy.

- Viscoelastic is then injected under the conjunctiva

- Triamcinolone or celectone chronodose injection subconjunctivally 0.1 ml behind the scleral flap at the end of the operation. 0.1 ml of garamycin (80 mg in 2 ml solution) are injected subconjunctivally in the lower fornix

For viscocanalostomy (VC) the steps are:

- Conjunctival dissection as for DS

- Application of MMC (0.2 mg/ml for 2-3 minutes) with the use of a few pieces of of a lasik shield arranged over a wide area under the conjunctiva.

- Superficial scleral flap creation as for DS

- Clear cornea phacoemulsification from a temporal approach with injectable intraocular lens insertion

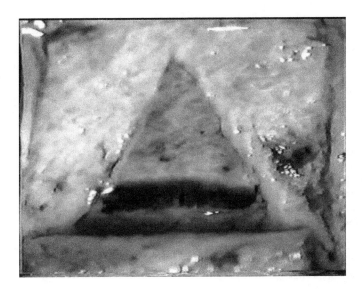

Figure 3. Deep sclerectomy site after excision of the deep scleral flap and peeling of the inner wall of the SC (courtesy of Prof Kozobolis)

- 10/0 nylon suture at the site of the main incision of the phacoemulsification

- Deep scleral flap formation as for DS

- Cannulation of the SC with the injection of high molecular weight viscoelastic device

- Unroofing of SC and dissection of deep peripheral corneal stroma from underlying Descemet's membrane

- Peeling of the inner wall of SC and juxtacanalicular trabeculum

- Excision of the deep scleral flap

- Tight suturing of the superficial flap to sclera with two 10/0 Nylon sutures

- Conjunctival closure with 10/0 nylon sutures.

Viscocanalostomy with or without the use of an implant has the same success rate [66]. One-site and two-site phaco-VC showed the same level of success [67].

5.7. Postoperative management

Topical steroids and antibiotics are given as in trabeculectomy. Again as for trabeculectomy antibiotics can be stopped after 4 weeks but steroids can be continued for 6 months or even longer at a low frequency. Cycloplegia is not necessary. As DS (and VC to a lesser extent) relies on a bleb formation for IOP control needling may be required if there is subconjunctival scarring or Tenon's cyst formation which are managed as described above. Tight sclera flap sutures are treated with argon laser suturolysis. Specifically for NPGS YAG laser puncture can be performed in case of iris prolapsed through the TDM with high IOP. The settings used are single pulsed shots, 3-5 mJoules through a gonioscopy lens. Pilocarpine 2% and argon laser iridoplasty can be used to pull away the iris from the site of incarceration. The settings for iridoplasty are 300-400µ spot size, 0.2 seconds exposure time, 300-400mWatt power through an iridectomy lens. If the IOP in the early or late postoperative period is thought to be due to poor aqueous filtration through the TDM, then YAG laser goniopuncture of the TDM can be tried. The settings are single pulsed shots, 4-6mJoules energy through a gonioscopy lens.

5.8. Outcomes

As opposed to phacotrabeculectomy, combined phaco-DS has better outcomes in terms of IOP control than DS alone [68]. Phacotrabeculectomy and phaco-DS showed no statistical difference in the IOP control although the phacotrabeculectomy groups tend to have lower IOP. Phaco-DS was the safer procedure in terms of complication rates [69,70].

Similarly viscocanalostomy offers slightly better hypotensive effect than phacoviscocanalostomy [71]. Compared to phacotrabeculectomy, phaco-VC offers similar IOP control in patients with primary open angle glaucoma. [72,73]

5.9. Complications

The complications of the combined cataract-glaucoma surgery include those of phacoemulsification and those of NPGS. The latter can be divided into intraoperative and postoperative.

- Intraoperative
    - Perforations of the TDM. Management: if small no further management is required. If they are large with iris prolapse a peripheral iridectomy should be carried out.
    - Hyphaema
- Postoperative
    - Early hypertony.
    - Causes:
        - retained viscoelastic. Management: observation, antiglaucoma drops, aspiration
        - haemorrhage in the scleral bed. Management: none required
        - Steroid response. Management: antiglaucoma drops, non-steroidal anti-inflammatory drugs
        - Rupture of the TDM with iris prolapse. Mechanism: rubbing of the eye, Valsalva's maneuver. Management: miotics, steroids, YAG laser of the prolapsed iris, argon laser iridoplasty, surgical removal of iris tissue
        - Pupillary block, aqueous misdirection, suprachoroidal haemorrhage. Management: as in trabeculectomy
    - Early hypotony
    - Causes:
        - Conjunctival wound leak. Management: suturing

- Ciliary body shutdown due to inflammation. Management: steroids

- MMC effect (toxic effect on the ciliary body)

- Hemorrhagic Descemet's membrane detachment [74] (fig 4,5)

- Ocular decompression retinopathy [75] (fig 6). It is caused by a sudden drop of the IOP during surgery. It is not exclusively seen in NPGS but also in penetrating glaucoma surgery, YAG laser iridotomy, and medical treatment for acute primary closure glaucoma (76,77)

- Late hypertony
  - Causes:
    - rupture of the TDM with iris prolapsed
    - Poor filtration through TDM. Management: YAG laser microperforations to TDM
    - Conjunctival scarring. Management: intensive topical steroids, subconjunctival injection of 5-FU/MMC
    - Bleb encapsulation. Management: bleb needling with 5-FU/MMC injections
- Late hypotony
  - Causes
    - Conjunctival wound leak
    - Ciliary body shutdown due to inflammation
    - MMC effect
- Blebitis and bleb related endophthalmitis

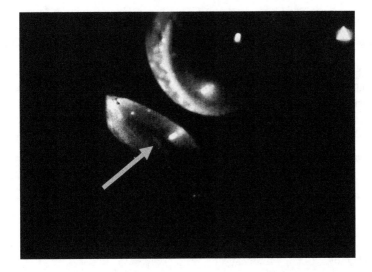

Figure 4. Hemorrhagic Descemet's membrane detachment (arrow) as seen through a Goldmann 4-mirror lens (courtesy of Prof Kozobolis)

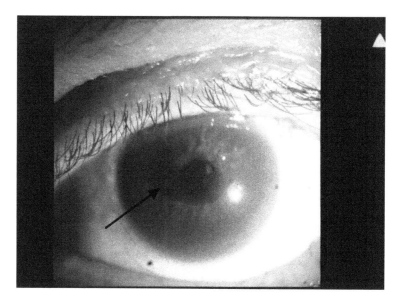

Figure 5. Hemorrhagic Descemet's membrane detachment 3 weeks postoperatively (arrow). The patient had a visual acuity of hand movements from 20/32 preoperatively. Six months after surgery the Descemet's membrane was completely re-atteched with a small residual scar. IOP control was excellent throughout the postoperative period (courtesy of Prof Kozobolis).

6. Combined phacoemulsification–glaucoma drainage devices (GDDs)

The first choice in the surgical management of glaucoma is a filtering operation. In some cases though, this type of surgical approach is thought to have low success rate. In these cases a GDD is the optimum choice.

6.1. Indications

The indications for this combined procedure are the presence of visually significant cataract in the presence of the following conditions:

- Failed trabeculectomy
- Neovascular glaucoma
- Primary and secondary congenital glaucoma
- Corneal grafts
- Traumatic glaucoma
- Extensive conjunctival scarring (e.g. buckle surgery)

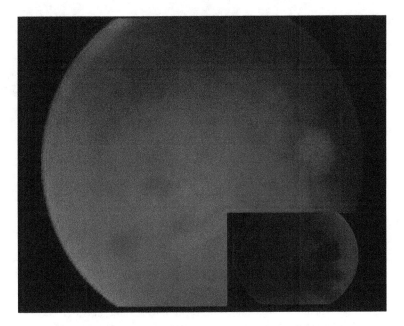

Figure 6. Decompression retinopathy. Insert: red free picture. This patient had a decrease of his visual acuity from 0.2 loMAR preoperatively to hand movements on the first postoperative day and the IOP dropped from 32 mmHg before surgery to 5 mmHg on the day after surgery. There was no leakage and the patient denied violent coughing or sneezing. The patient was prescribed the standard postoperative topical medication. An intravenous fluorescein angiogram did not show any evidence of central retinal vein occlusion. The visual acuity improved to preoperative level 3 months after surgery and the retinal haemorrhages gradually disappeared. IOP ranged from 7-14 mmHg without any topical antiglaucoma drops (courtesy of Prof Kozobolis)

- Primary surgery in open angle glaucoma (Ahmed GDD)

6.2. Choice of GDD

When deciding which GDD to use the surgeon should have in mind that:

- Valved GDDs allow unidirectional flow with low opening pressure and do not require ligating suture

- Non valved GDDs require ligation of the lumen with 7/0 or 8/0 Vicryl suture and/or occlusion of the lumen with 3/0 supramid suture (nylon braided)

- Size of plate: the larger the plate the larger the fibrous capsule around the plate and filtration area. However numerous studies have shown that in the long term the larger plates do not produce significantly lower intraocular pressures [78-79]

- Plate material: silicone plates seem to do better than the polypropylene ones with lower complication rate (Tenon's cyst formation) [80-84].

6.3. Antimetabolites and anti–VEGF

There is conflicting evidence as to whether MMC and bevacizumab improve the success rate of Ahmed GDD. Mahdy et al [85] reported that both the application of MMC and injection of bevacizumab around the footplate of the GDD at the end of the operation improve the hypotensive effect. Alvarado et al [86] found that the use of high concentrations and application time of MMC also offer better hypotensive effect. On the other several other authors have reported that the intraoperative use of MMC did not improve the results of the GDD implantation [87-90].

6.4. Surgical technique

The surgical technique described below applies mainly to the Ahmed GDD as this is the GDD that we use.

- 7/0 Vicryl corneal traction suture 4 mm from the limbus at the quadrant of the GDD insertion (optional)

- Conjunctival and Tenon's dissection (fornix based, supero-temporal quadrant preferably). Limbal peritomy extends for 3-4 o'clock hours. Relieving cuts are made perpendicular to the limbus in order to achieve better exposure of the sclera.

- When using large plate GDDs lateral/medial rectus muscles and superior rectus need to be isolated with brindle 4/0 silk sutures

- Fixate plate on the sclera wit 8/0 nylon sutures. The plate is fixated 8mm from the limbus and the suture needles are passed through the holes at the anterior edge of the plate

- Prime valved GDDs. The GDDs are primed by irrigating BSS with a 30G blunt canula from the tip of the tube. BSS should exit at the proximal end of the tube

- Trim tube. The surgeon trims the tube with scissors allowing about 3 mm of the tube length to enter in the anterior chamber in front of the iris

- Preplace tube fixation suture (9/0 silk) on sclera

- Preplace patch graft sutures (8/0 nylon) on sclera. Two sutures are used one at each side of the graft. Preplacing the sutures reduces the period of hypotony during the GDD insertion. The patch graft may be sclera, pericardium, cornea, fascia lata or dura.

- Do clear cornea phacoemulsification (away from the area of GDD insertion, suture main incision)

- Create track for the tube with 22 or 23G needle. The needle is bent at 90° at two places with the bevel of the tip of the needle facing upwards. The needle is inserted 1 mm behind the limbus at a plane parallel to the iris. The needle is mounted on a viscoelastic syringe. Viscoelastic can be injected as the needle is withdrawn in order to keep the tract open and facilitate the tube insertion

- Insert tube in anterior chamber. The tube is grasped with serrated forceps near the tip and pushed along the needle track. It may need to be grasped several times until it is inserted

- Tie the tube fixation suture. The suture must not occlude the lumen of the tube

- Tie patch graft sutures

- Suture Tenon's capsule and conjunctiva. The conjunctiva is first sutured at the limbus at its two corners. The relaxing incisions are sutured with running sutures. Finally the anterior edge of the conjunctiva is sutured to the limbus with two horizontal mattress sutures. We use 10/0 nylon for this step of the procedure

- Supramid suture must protrude under the conjunctiva so that it can be removed later in the postoperative period

6.5. Complications

The complications of the combined cataract-glaucoma surgery include those of phacoemulsification and those of the GDDs.

GDD complications

- Hypotony(more likely with non valved GDDs)
  - Causes:
    - incomplete obstruction of the non valved GDDs. Management: resuturing
    - Leakage around the tube. Management: repositioning of the tube
    - inflammation
- Hypertensive phase (most common with Ahmed GDDs).

  Mechanism: formation of fibrous capsule around the plate. Management: antiglaucoma drops, ocular massage, needling with 5-FU, removal of GDD

- Tube occlusion

  Causes: blood, fibrin, vitreous, iris. Management: removal of the agent that causes the obstruction with YAG laser or surgically.

- Tube/graft erosion through conjunctiva. Management: covering of the tube with donor sclera.
- Tube touching corneal endothelium. Management: repositioning of the tube
- Retraction of the GDD. Management: repositioning of the GDD
- Endothelial decompensation
- Diplopia (large plate GDDs). Management: prisms, strabismus surgery, removal of GDD.
- Endophthalmitis

6.6. Postoperative management

Topical antibiotic and steroids are given as for trabeculectomy. Antibiotics can be stopped one month postoperatively but steroids will need to be continued for longer. Cycloplegia is given for 2-3 weeks. Ahmed GDDs are renowned for their hypertensive phase which happens after

3-6 weeks as fibrous tissue is forming around the plate. The IOP must be lowered with topical antiglaucoma medication or even acetozolamide tablets. Needling of the fibrous capsule with 30G needle may be tried with injection of dexamethasone and 5FU as for trabeculectomy.

6.7. Outcomes

The combined surgery does not seem to adversely affect the hypotensive effect of the GDD [91].

7. Combined phacoemulsification–Ex-PRESS GDD

The Ex-PRESS GDD works differently compared to the GDDs described above. It is a miniature stainless steel non valved GDD with 0.4mm external diameter and 50 or 200 μm internal diameter depending on the model. It has a length of 2.4 – 3.0 mm, it is safe in magnetic fields up to 3 Tesla [92,93] and does seem to interfere with the quality of the MRI images of the orbit [94].

7.1. Indications

• Open angle glaucomas

• In case of narrow angles there may not be enough room to fit the mini implant

• Is not the best option in congenital glaucomas as it is a new procedure and the concomitant use of antimetabolites may cause problems in the long run in young patients.

7.2. Aqueous humor dynamics in Ex–PRESS GDD

The Ex-PRESS GDD is an alternative to trabeculectomy as it only replaces the internal ostium and negates the need for a peripheral iridectomy. The aqueous flows through the GDD in the subconjunctival/sub-Tenon's space and forms a filtering bleb.

7.3. Antimetabolites

The insertion of the Ex-PRESS GDD can be augmented with the intraoperative application of MMC in order to reduce conjunctival scarring and improve bleb survival

7.4. Corticosteroids

As with trabeculectomy the authors augment the operation with the injection of 0.1 ml of triamcinolone under the conjunctiva behind the scleral flap at the end of the operation. Standard postoperative care includes the use of topical steroids and antibiotics.

7.5. Surgical technique

• The initial steps for the combined phaco- Ex-PRESS GDD procedure are the same as for trabeculectomy up to the creation of the track for the insertion of the mini shunt

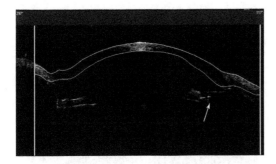

Figure 7. Ex-PRESS GDD indenting the iris (arrow) without any adverse effects and excellent IOP control(courtesy of Prof Kozobolis)

• Ex-PRESS inserted at the blue transition zone between clear cornea and sclera (corresponds to juxtacanalicular meshwork) with the use of a 25G needle. The direction of the needle must be parallel to the iris plane. The needle is advanced until it is clearly seen in the anterior chamber

• Tying of the scleral flap releasable sutures (more sutures can be used according to the surgeon's discretion).

• Conjunctival closure with 10/0 nylon sutures as in trabeculectomy.

• Triamcinolone injection subconjunctivally 0.1 ml behind the scleral flap at the end of the operation.

7.6. Postoperative management

As the insertion of the Ex-PRESS GDD is a small trabeculectomy the postoperative management is the same as for trabeculectomy.

7.7. Complications

As the Ex-PRESS mini GDD is a modification of trabeculectomy and the aqueous dynamics are similar the complications from its insertion are similar to that of trabeculectomy. Complications specific to the technique include obstruction of the GDD by blood, fibrin and vitreous. The device may also touch the iris and can be repositioned via another track (fig 7). The track can be done under the same sclera flap next to the initial one. Mal-positioned devices do not need to be re-inserted if they are symptom free and offer adequate hypotensive effect (fig 8). The Ex-PRESS mini shunt may be blocked by fibrin, blood or vitreous. YAG laser is an excellent tool which can be used to remove the blockage [95].

7.8. Outcomes

The Ex-Press GDD is at least as effective as TM in terms of long term IOP control and number of postoperative antiglaucoma drops. It also has lower complication rate compared to

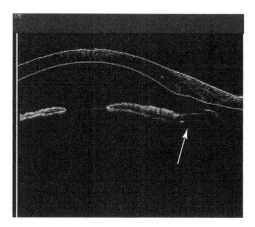

Figure 8. Ex-PRESS GDD (arrow) inserted through a patent peripheral iridectomy in posterior chamber with excellent IOP control (courtesy of Prof Kozobolis)

trabeculectomy [96-101].The combined phaco-Ex-PRESS operation has the hypotensive effect as the simple insertion of the device [102].

8. New techniques

The aim of the procedures is to enhance the normal outflow of aqueous via the conventional and uveoscleral pathways without the formation of a filtering bleb. The Trabektome, the Eyepass and the Glaukos iStent require access to SC trough the trabeculum and can be combined with phacoemulsification which by the removal of a bulky cataractous crystalline lens facilitates access to the anterior chamber angle.

8.1. Indications

The indications of the new techniques is mild to moderate open angle glaucoma

8.2. Surgical technique

The micro-implants described below are inserted after the completion of standard phacoemulsification

9. Canaloplasty

9.1. Surgical technique

• Conjunctival dissection

- Formation of a 5×5 mm superficial scleral flap at 50% of sclera thickness
- Formation of a 4×4 mm deep scleral flap extending into clear cornea to create a Descemet's window as for DS
- Clear cornea phacoemulsification from a temporal approach with injectable intraocular lens insertion
- Excision of the deep scleral flap
- Insertion of a microcatheter in one of the two cut ends of Schlemm's canal (iTrack 250A)
- The microcatheter is pushed around SC with injection of sodium hyaluronate in order to dilate the canal and create microruptures in the wall.
- The microcatheter has a light at its tip so that the surgeon can follow it as it is driven around SC
- When the tip of the microcatheter emerges at the other cut end of SC a 10/0 Nylon suture is tied on the tip and the microcatheter is pulled back
- When the tip of the microcatheter emerges from the cut end of SC the two ends are tied together to provide moderate tension on the canal.
- The superficial flap is tied securely to the sclera with 10/0 Nylon
- Conjunctiva is sutured with 10/0 Nylon

9.2. Outcomes

Combined phaco-canalostomy provides slightly better hypotensive effect and less antiglaucoma drops than canalostomy alone [103,104]. Compared to trabeculectomy it offers lower but not statistically significant hypotensive effect and requires more antiglaucoma medication than trabeculectomy [105].

9.3. Complications

The most common complications are hyphaema, peripheral anterior synechiae, Descemet membrane detachment

10. Solx gold microshunt (GMS)

The GMS is a flat-plate non valved drainage device which is inserted in the suprachoroidal space and increases uveoscleral outflow. It is made of 24 karat gold and its dimensions are 3.2 mm wide, 5.2 mm long and 44μm thick. The aqueous enters the device from the proximal side which contains 60 holes 100 μm each. The device contains 10 open and 9 closed channels (width of lumen 24μm and height 50μm) and at the distal end the fluid exits in the suprachoroidal space via a grid of 117 holes on either side. The proximal end of the GMS contains 12 additional channels and the distal end 10 channels 50 μm each

10.1. Surgical technique [106]

• Conjunctival dissection at the limbus

• Full thickness scleral incision 2.5 mm behind the limbus down to the ciliary body. Anterior chamber is entered at 90% of the scleral thickness with a crescent knife

• Posterior dissection to expose the suprachoroidal space with a blunt cannula for 4-5 mm

• The anterior part of the GMS is placed in the anterior chamber and the posterior in the suprachoroidal space

• The implant is pushed posteriorly with an insulin needle so that 1-1.5 mm of the proximal end is in the anterior chamber

• Sclera is closed with 7/0 Vicryl sutures

• Conjunctiva is sutured with 10/0 Nylon sutures

10.2. Outcomes

Figus et al [107] reported 67% qualified success at 2 years. Melamed et al [106] reported 79% success rate with or without medication after a mean follow up period of 11.7 months

10.3. Complications

Hyphaema, choroidal effusions, bullous keratopathy due to contact of the implant with the endothelium, exudative retinal detachment due to overfiltration

11. Glaukos iStent

The iStent is an L shaped titanium device 1mm long with an internal lumen diameter of 120 μm. It is inserted in the SC following phacoemulsification. The most common complication is stent malposition and obstruction by blood, vitreous, fibrin.

11.1. Outcomes

Samuelson et al [108] reported that combined phaco-iStent provided better hypotensive effect at one year than simple phacoemulsification which is statistically significant. Craven et al [109] also support this finding with phaco-iStent which offers better IOP control at 2 years than phacoemulsification.

12. Trabektome

Trabektome is a foot switch operated handpiece which ablates the trabeculum and inner wall of SC and can follow phacoemulsification with a temporal approach. If the anterior chamber angle is wide enough the ablation can take place before cataract extraction through the main incision. The Trabektome's handpiece has an aspiration port and an electrocautery-ablation system. The handpiece is driven along the nasal angle and treats an area of 60°-120° of trabeculum

12.1. Outcomes

Ting et al [110] reported that Trabektome controls IOP better in eyes with pseudoexfoliation glaucoma than primary open angle glaucoma and has more profound effect when combined with phacoemulsification.

13. Aquashunt

The Aquashunt device is placed in the suprachoroidal space and aims to facilitate aqueous outflow via the uveoscleral pathway. Instead a multiple small channels it has one large channel. A phase I multicenter trial is being conducted.

14. Eyepass

The Eyepass intracanalicular stent is a Y-shaped 1 mm long silicone tube that can be inserted in the SC following phacoemulsification. The two arms of the tube are inserted in the SC and the dual-bonded end protrudes in the anterior chamber.

14.1. Surgical technique [111]

- Conjunctival dissection at the limbus

- Formation of a superficial scleral flap (as in NPGS)

- Clear cornea phacoemulsification away from the area of the scleral flap

- Creation of the deep scleral flap with unroofing of the SC

- Dilatation of the SC with viscoelastic device (sodium hyaluronate 1%)

- Insertion of the two arms of Eyepass in the SC

- Insertion of the common stem of the device in the anterior chamber through a paracentesis 1 mm in front of the trabeculum

- Watertight suturing of the scleral flap with 10/0 Nylon sutures

- Conjunctiva closed with 10/0 Nylon sutures

14.2. Complications

The most serious complication is the perforation of the trabeculum during insertion of the arms of the device and conversion to trabeculectomy.

14.3. Outcomes

Dietlein et al [111] reported good hypotensive effect with fewer antiglaucoma drops of the Eyepass combined with phacoemulsification in patients with pseudoexfoliation and primary open angle glaucoma.

15. CyPass

The Cypass is a polyamide implant 6mm long with a 300 μm diameter that is inserted ab interno in the suprachoroidal space with a specially designed inserter. It is inserted through the main incision of cataract surgery following clear cornea phacoemulsification [112]. Lanchulev et al reported IOP reduction from 22.9 mmHg to 16.2 mmHg after 6 months in eyes that underwent phacoemulsification and Cypass insertion [113]. Craven et al reported that the most common adverse effects are: hyphaema, persistent inflammation, branch retinal vein occlusion and exacerbation of diabetic macular oedema [114].

16. Ciliary body endophotocoagulation (ECP)

Photocoagulation of the ciliary body processes is done by a 810 nm semiconductor diode laser. The endoscope carries the viewing system, the laser system and the light source. The procedure can be applied via a pars plana approach or from corneal incision. The treatment is applied over 360°. When it is delivered through a corneal incision it can follow phacoemulsification as the removal of the crystalline lens offers easier access to the ciliary processes. The probe is pushed forward between the intraocular lens implant and the iris

16.1. Outcomes

Phaco-ECP provides good control of the IOP in early/moderate glaucoma over time with no ECP related complications [115]. This study also suggests that phaco-ECP offers an additional hypotensive effect to phacoemulsification alone. Lima et al compared ECP with Ahmed GDD in the treatment of refractory glaucoma and found no differences in the success rate. Ahmed GDD had a higher complication rate than ECP [116].

17. Summary

Phaco-trabeculectomy remains the standard procedure for the management of coexisting cataract and glaucoma. Newer techniques have been developed in order to avoid entering the eye and provide a more controlled reduction of the IOP. The use of antifibrotic agents have improved the survival of these procedures but also increased the incidence of complications. On the other hand the development of the newer antiglaucoma drops gave more options to the ophthalmologists for the medical management of glaucoma but have adversely affected the outcome of the antiglaucoma surgery.

The glaucoma drainage implants retain their place as a useful tool in many forms of severe glaucoma where the penetrating and non-penetrating procedures are likely to fail. The Ex-PRESS mini implant is a penetrating procedure but has a better safety profile and equal hypotensive effect to trabeculectomy.

Current research aims to the development of miniature devices that will facilitate the drainage of aqueous via the physiological pathways without leading to aqueous accumulation under the external coatings of the eye.

Author details

Vassilis Kozobolis, Aristeidis Konstantinidis* and Georgios Labiris

*Address all correspondence to: aristeidiskon@hotmail.com

Eye department, University Hospital of Alexandroupolis, Alexandroupolis, Greece

References

[1] Foster, P. J, Buhrmann, R, Quigley, H. A, & Johnson, G. J. The definition and classification of glaucoma in prevalence surveys. Br J Ophthalmol. (2002). Feb;, 86(2), 238-42.

[2] Quigley, H. A, & Broman, A. T. The number of people with glaucoma worldwide in 2010 and 2020.Br J Ophthalmol. (2006). Mar;, 90(3), 262-7.

[3] Quigley, H. A. Number of people with glaucoma worldwide. Br J Ophthalmol. (1996). May;, 80(5), 389-93.

[4] Davanger, M, Ringvold, A, & Blika, S. The probability of having glaucoma at different IOP levels. Acta Ophthalmol (Copenh). (1991). Oct;, 69(5), 565-8.

[5] Boateng, W. Economics of surgery worldwide. Developing countries. Glaucoma Saunders. Philadelphia. , 1, 13.

[6] Migdal, C, Gregory, W, & Hitchings, R. Long-term functional outcome after early surgery compared with laser and medicine in open-angle glaucoma. Ophthalmology. (1994). Oct;, 101(10), 1651-6.

[7] Lichter, P. R, Musch, D. C, Gillespie, B. W, Guire, K. E, Janz, N. K, & Wren, P. A. Mills RP; CIGTS Study Group. Interim clinical outcomes in the Collaborative Initial Glaucoma Treatment Study comparing initial treatment randomized to medications or surgery. Ophthalmology. (2001). Nov;, 108(11), 1943-53.

[8] Chen, T. C, Wilensky, J. T, & Viana, M. A. Long-term follow-up of initially successful trabeculectomy. Ophthalmology. (1997). Jul;, 104(7), 1120-5.

[9] Nouri-mahdavi, K, Brigatti, L, Weitzman, M, & Caprioli, J. Outcomes of trabeculectomy for primary open-angle glaucoma. Ophthalmology. (1995). Dec;, 102(12), 1760-9.

[10] Keenan, T. D, Wotton, C. J, & Goldacre, M. J. Recent trends in the rate of trabeculectomy in England. Eye (Lond). (2011). Sep;25(9).

[11] Whittaker, K. W, Gillow, J. T, & Cunliffe, I. A. Is the role of trabeculectomy in glaucoma management changing? Eye (Lond). (2001). Aug;15(Pt 4):449-52.

[12] Strutton, D. R, & Walt, J. G. Trends in glaucoma surgery before and after the introduction of new topical glaucoma pharmacotherapies. J Glaucoma. (2004). Jun;, 13(3), 221-6.

[13] Rachmiel, R, Trope, G. E, Chipman, M. L, Gouws, P, & Buys, Y. M. Laser trabeculoplasty trends with the introduction of new medical treatments and selective laser trabeculoplasty. J Glaucoma. (2006). Aug;, 15(4), 306-9.

[14] Knox, F. A, Barry, M, Mcgowan, B, & Brien, O. C. The rising cost of glaucoma drugs in Ireland 1996-2003. Br J Ophthalmol. (2006). Feb;, 90(2), 162-5.

[15] Shingleton, B. J, Pasternack, J. J, Hung, J. W, Donoghue, O, & Three, M. W. and five year changes in intraocular pressures after clear corneal phacoemulsification in open angle glaucoma patients, glaucoma suspects, and normal patients. J Glaucoma. (2006). Dec;, 15(6), 494-8.

[16] Cimetta, D. J, & Cimetta, A. C. Intraocular pressure changes after clear corneal phacoemulsification in nonglaucomatous pseudoexfoliation syndrome. Eur J Ophthalmol. (2008). Jan-Feb;, 18(1), 77-81.

[17] Brig JKS PariharLt Col Jaya Kaushik, Surg Lt Cdr AS Parihar and Ashwini KS Parihar. Combined approach to co-existing glaucoma and cataract. In Pinakin Gunvant (ed). Glaucoma-Current clinical and research aspects. Rijeka: InTech; (2011). , 275.

[18] Husain, R, Liang, S, Foster, P. J, Gazzard, G, Bunce, C, Chew, P. T, Oen, F. T, Khaw, P. T, Seah, S. K, & Aung, T. Cataract surgery after trabeculectomy: the effect on trabeculectomy function. Arch Ophthalmol. (2012). Feb;, 130(2), 165-70.

[19] Liu, H. N, Li, X, Nie, Q. Z, & Chen, X. L. Efficacy and tolerability of one-site versus two-site phacotrabeculectomy: a meta-analysis. Int J Ophthalmol. (2010). , 3(3), 264-8.

[20] Nassiri, N, Nassiri, N, Mohammadi, B, & Rahmani, . . Comparison of 2 surgical techniques in phacotrabeculectomy: 1 site versus 2 sites. Eur J Ophthalmol. 2010 Mar-Apr;20(2):316-26.

[21] Gdih, G. A, Yuen, D, Yan, P, Sheng, L, Jin, Y. P, & Buys, Y. M. Meta-analysis of 1-versus 2-Site Phacotrabeculectomy. Ophthalmology. (2011). Jan;, 118(1), 71-6.

[22] Wells, A. P, Cordeiro, M. F, Bunce, C, & Khaw, P. T. Cystic bleb formation and related complications in limbus- versus fornix-based conjunctival flaps in pediatric and young adult trabeculectomy with mitomycin C. Ophthalmology. (2003). Nov;, 110(11), 2192-7.

[23] Tezel, G, Kolker, A. E, Kass, M. A, & Wax, M. B. Comparative results of combined procedures for glaucoma and cataract: II. Limbus-based versus fornix-based conjunctival flaps. Ophthalmic Surg Lasers. (1997). Jul;, 28(7), 551-7.

[24] Kozobolis, V. P, Siganos, C. S, Christodoulakis, E. V, Lazarov, N. P, Koutentaki, M. G, & Pallikaris, I. G. Two-site phacotrabeculectomy with intraoperative mitomycin-C: fornix- versus limbus-based conjunctival opening in fellow eyes. J Cataract Refract Surg. (2002). Oct;, 28(10), 1758-62.

[25] Solus, J. F, Jampel, H. D, Tracey, P. A, Gilbert, D. L, Loyd, T. L, Jefferys, J. L, & Quigley, H. A. Comparison of limbus-based and fornix-based trabeculectomy: success, bleb-related complications, and bleb morphology. Ophthalmology. (2012). Apr;, 119(4), 703-11.

[26] The Advanced Glaucoma Intervention Study (AGIS): 11Risk factors for failure of trabeculectomy and argon laser trabeculoplasty. AGIS Investigators. Am J Ophthalmol. (2002). Oct;, 134(4), 481-98.

[27] Scott, I. U, Greenfield, D. S, Schiffman, J, Nicolela, M. T, Rueda, J. C, Tsai, J. C, & Palmberg, P. F. Outcomes of primary trabeculectomy with the use of adjunctive mitomycin. Arch Ophthalmol. (1998). Mar;, 116(3), 286-91.

[28] Stürmer, J, Broadway, D. C, & Hitchings, R. A. Young patient trabeculectomy. Assessment of risk factors for failure. Ophthalmology. (1993). Jun;, 100(6), 928-39.

[29] Broadway, D, & Grierson, I. Hitchings R Racial differences in the results of glaucoma filtration surgery: are racial differences in the conjunctival cell profile important? Br J Ophthalmol. (1994). Jun;, 78(6), 466-75.

[30] Jacobi, P. C, Dietlein, T. S, & Krieglstein, G. K. Primary trabeculectomy in young adults: long-term clinical results and factors influencing the outcome. Ophthalmic Surg Lasers. (1999). Sep-Oct;, 30(8), 637-46.

[31] Flach, A. J. Does medical treatment influence the success of trabeculectomy? Trans Am Ophthalmol Soc. (2004). discussion 223-4, 102, 219-23.

[32] Lavin, M. J, Wormald, R. P, Migdal, C. S, & Hitchings, R. A. The influence of prior therapy on the success of trabeculectomy. Arch Ophthalmol. (1990). Nov; , 108(11), 1543-8.

[33] Broadway, D. C, Grierson, I, & Hitchings, R. A. Local effects of previous conjunctival incisional surgery and the subsequent outcome of filtration surgery. Am J Ophthalmol. (1998). Jun;, 125(6), 805-18.

[34] Olali, C, Rotchford, A. P, & King, A. J. Outcome of repeat trabeculectomies. Clin Experiment Ophthalmol. (2011). Sep-Oct;, 39(7), 658-64.

[35] Cankaya, A. B, & Elgin, U. Comparison of the outcome of repeat trabeculectomy with adjunctive mitomycin C and initial trabeculectomy. Korean J Ophthalmol. (2011). Dec;, 25(6), 401-8.

[36] Mietz, H, Raschka, B, & Krieglstein, G. K. Risk factors for failures of trabeculectomies performed without antimetabolites. Br J Ophthalmol. (1999). Jul;, 83(7), 814-21.

[37] Hugkulstone, C. E, Smith, L. F, & Vernon, S. A. Trabeculectomy in diabetic patients with glaucoma. Eye (1993). , 7, 502-506.

[38] Joshi, A. B, Parrish, R. K, & Feuer, W. F. (2002). survey of the American glaucoma society: Practice preferences for glaucoma surgery and antifbrotic use. J Glaucoma 2005;, 14, 172-174.

[39] Lin, Z. J, Li, Y, Cheng, J. W, & Lu, X. H. Intraoperative mitomycin C versus intraoperative 5-fluorouracil for trabeculectomy: a systematic review and meta-analysis. J Ocul Pharmacol Ther. (2012). Apr;, 28(2), 166-73.

[40] Wilkins, M, Indar, A, & Wormald, R. Intra-operative mitomycin C for glaucoma surgery. Cochrane Database Syst Rev. (2005). Oct 19;(4):CD002897.

[41] Five year follow-up of the fluorouracil filtering surgery studyThe fluorouracil filtering surgery study group. Am J Ophthalmol (1996). , 121, 349-366.

[42] The Fluorouracil Filtering Surgery Group: fluorouracil filtering surgery study one year follow upAm J Ophthamlol (2001). , 12, 143-148.

[43] Beckers, H. J, Kinders, K. C, & Webers, C. A. Five-year results of trabeculectomy with mitomycin C. Graefes Arch Clin Exp Ophthalmol. (2003). Feb;, 241(2), 106-10.

[44] Zacharia, P. T, Deppermann, S. R, & Schuman, J. S. Ocular hypotony after trabeculectomy with mitomycin C. Am J Ophthalmol. (1993). Sep 15;, 116(3), 314-26.

[45] Higginbotham, E. J, Stevens, R. K, Musch, D. C, Karp, K. O, Lichter, P. R, Bergstrom, T. J, & Skuta, G. L. Bleb-related endophthalmitis after trabeculectomy with mitomycin C. Ophthalmology. (1996). Apr;, 103(4), 650-6.

[46] Araujo, S. V, Spaeth, G. L, Roth, S. M, & Starita, R. J. A ten-year follow-up on a prospective, randomized trial of postoperative corticosteroids after trabeculectomy. Ophthalmology. (1995). Dec;, 102(12), 1753-9.

[47] Lavin, M. J, Wormald, R. P, Migdal, C. S, & Hitchings, R. A. The influence of prior therapy on the success of trabeculectomy. Arch Ophthalmol. (1990). Nov;, 108(11), 1543-8.

[48] Broadway, D. C, Grierson, I, Brien, O, & Hitchings, C. RA. Adverse effects of topical antiglaucoma medication. II. The outcome of filtration surgery. Arch Ophthalmol. (1994). Nov;, 112(11), 1446-54.

[49] Breusegem, C, Spielberg, L, Van Ginderdeuren, R, Vandewalle, E, & Renier, C. Van de Veire S, Fieuws S, Zeyen T, Stalmans I. Preoperative non steroidal anti-inflammatory drug or steroid and outcomes after trabeculectomy: a randomized controlled trial. Ophthalmology. (2010). Jul;, 117(7), 1324-30.

[50] Tham, C. C, Li, F. C, Leung, D. Y, Kwong, Y. Y, Yick, D. W, Chi, C. C, & Lam, D. S. Intrableb triamcinolone acetonide injection after bleb-forming filtration surgery (trabeculectomy, phacotrabeculectomy, and trabeculectomy revision by needling): a pilot study. Eye (Lond). (2006). Dec;, 20(12), 1484-6.

[51] Kahook, M. Y, Camejo, L, & Noecker, R. J. Trabeculectomy with intraoperative retrobulbar triamcinolone acetonide. Clin Ophthalmol. (2009). , 3, 29-31.

[52] Yuki, K, Shiba, D, Kimura, I, Ohtake, Y, & Tsubota, K. Trabeculectomy with or without intraoperative sub-tenon injection of triamcinolone acetonide in treating secondary glaucoma. Am J Ophthalmol. (2009). Jun;, 147(6), 1055-60.

[53] Nilforushan, N, Yadgari, M, Kish, S. K, & Nassiri, N. Subconjunctival bevacizumab versus mitomycin C adjunctive to trabeculectomy.Am J Ophthalmol. (2012). Feb;, 153(2), 352-357.

[54] Sedghipour, M. R, Mostafaei, A, & Taghavi, Y. Low-dose subconjunctival bevacizumab to augment trabeculectomy for glaucoma. Clin Ophthalmol. (2011). , 5, 797-800.

[55] Friedman, D. S, Jampel, H. D, Lubomski, L. H, Kempen, J. H, Quigley, H, Congdon, N, Levkovitch-verbin, H, Robinson, K. A, & Bass, E. B. Surgical strategies for coexisting glaucoma and cataract: an evidence-based update. Ophthalmology. (2002). Oct;, 109(10), 1902-13.

[56] Tripathi, R. C, Tripathi, B. J, Park, J. K, Quaranta, L, Steinspair, K, Lehman, E, & Ernest, J. T. Intracameral tissue plasminogen activator for resolution of fibrin clots after glaucoma filtering procedures. Am J Ophthalmol. (1991). Feb 15;, 111(2), 247-8.

[57] Seah, S. K. Prata JA Jr, Minckler DS, Baerveldt G, Lee PP, Heuer DK. Hypotony following trabeculectomy. J Glaucoma. (1995). Apr;, 4(2), 73-9.

[58] Bindlish, R, Condon, G. P, Schlosser, J. D, Antonio, D, Lauer, J, Lehrer, K. B, & Efficacy, R. and safety of mitomycin-C in primary trabeculectomy: five-year follow-up. Ophthalmology. (2002). Jul;discussion 1341-2., 109(7), 1336-41.

[59] Costa, V. P, & Arcieri, E. S. Hypotony maculopathy [review].Acta Ophthalmol Scand (2007). , 85, 586-597.

[60] Mietz, H. The toxicology of mitomycin C on the ciliary body. Curr Opin Ophthalmol. (1996). Apr;, 7(2), 72-9.

[61] Nuyts, R. M, Greve, E. L, Geijssen, H. C, & Langerhorst, C. T. Treatment of hypotonous maculopathy after trabeculectomy with mitomycin C. Am J Ophthalmol. (1994). Sep 15;, 118(3), 322-31.

[62] Lüke, C, Dietlein, T. S, Jacobi, P. C, Konen, W, & Krieglstein, G. K. Ophthalmology.Risk profile of deep sclerectomy for treatment of refractory congenital glaucomas. (2002). Jun; , 109(6), 1066-71.

[63] Noureddin, B. N, Haibi, C. P, Cheikha, A, & Bashshur, Z. F. Viscocanalostomy versus trabeculotomy ab externo in primary congenital glaucoma: 1-year follow-up of a prospective controlled pilot study. Br J Ophthalmol. (2006). Oct;, 90(10), 1281-5.

[64] Kay, J. S, Mitchell, R, & Miller, J. Dilation and Probing of Schlemm's Canal and Viscocanalostomy in Pediatric Glaucoma. J Pediatr Ophthalmol Strabismus. (2011). Jan-Feb;doi:, 48(1), 30-7.

[65] Yarangümeli, A, Köz, O. G, Alp, M. N, Elhan, A. H, & Kural, G. Viscocanalostomy with mitomycin-C: a preliminary study. Eur J Ophthalmol. (2005). Mar-Apr;, 15(2), 202-8.

[66] Anand, N, & Atherley, C. Deep sclerectomy augmented with mitomycin C. Eye (Lond). (2005). Apr;, 19(4), 442-50.

[67] Lüke, C, Dietlein, T. S, Jacobi, P. C, Konen, W, & Krieglstein, G. K. A prospective randomised trial of viscocanalostomy with and without implantation of a reticulated hyaluronic acid implant (SKGEL) in open angle glaucoma. Br J Ophthalmol. (2003). May;, 87(5), 599-603.

[68] Gimbel, H. V, Penno, E. E, & Ferensowicz, M. Combined cataract surgery, intraocular lens implantation, and viscocanalostomy. J Cataract Refract Surg. (1999). Oct;, 25(10), 1370-5.

[69] Eliseo, D, Pastena, D, Longanesi, B, Grisanti, L, & Negrini, F. V. Comparison of deep sclerectomy with implant and combined glaucoma surgery. Ophthalmologica. (2003). May-Jun;, 217(3), 208-11.

[70] Cillino, S. Di Pace F, Casuccio A, Calvaruso L, Morreale D, Vadalà M, Lodato G. Deep sclerectomy versus punch trabeculectomy with or without phacoemulsification: a randomized clinical trial. J Glaucoma. (2004). Dec;, 13(6), 500-6.

[71] Funnell, C. L, Clowes, M, & Anand, N. Combined cataract and glaucoma surgery with mitomycin C: phacoemulsification-trabeculectomy compared to phacoemulsification-deepsclerectomy.Br J Ophthalmol. (2005). Jun;, 89(6), 694-8.

[72] Wishart, M. S, Shergill, T, & Porooshani, H. Viscocanalostomy and phacoviscocanalostomy: long-term results. J Cataract Refract Surg. (2002). May;, 28(5), 745-51.

[73] Tanito, M, Park, M, Nishikawa, M, Ohira, A, & Chihara, E. Comparison of surgical outcomes of combined viscocanalostomy and cataract surgery with combined trabeculotomy and cataract surgery. Am J Ophthalmol. (2002). Oct;, 134(4), 513-20.

[74] Kobayashi, H, & Kobayashi, K. Randomized comparison of the intraocular pressure-lowering effect of phacoviscocanalostomy and phacotrabeculectomy. Ophthalmology. (2007). May;, 114(5), 909-14.

[75] Kozobolis, V. P, Christodoulakis, E. V, Siganos, C. S, & Pallikaris, I. G. Hemorrhagic Descemet's membrane detachment as a complication of deep sclerectomy: a case report.J Glaucoma. (2001). Dec;, 10(6), 497-500.

[76] Kozobolis, V. P, Kalogianni, E, Katsanos, A, Dardabounis, D, Koukoula, S, & Labiris, G. Ocular decompression retinopathy after deep sclerectomy with mitomycin C in an eye with exfoliation glaucoma. Eur J Ophthalmol. (2011). May-Jun;, 21(3), 324-7.

[77] Alwitry, A, Khan, K, Rotchford, A, Zaman, A. G, & Vernon, S. A. Severe decompression retinopathy after medical treatment of acute primary angle closure. Br J Ophthalmol. (2007). Jan;91(1):121

[78] Landers, J, & Craig, J. Decompression retinopathy and corneal oedema following Nd:YAG laser peripheral iridotomy. Clin. Experiment Ophthalmol. (2006). Mar;, 34(2), 182-4.

[79] Molteno, A. C, Bevin, T. H, Herbison, P, & Houliston, M. J. Otago glaucoma surgery outcome study: long-term follow-up of cases of primary glaucoma with additional risk factors drained by Molteno implants. Ophthalmology. (2001). Dec;, 108(12), 2193-200.

[80] Britt, M. T. LaBree LD, Lloyd MA, Minckler DS, Heuer DK, Baerveldt G, Varma R. Randomized clinical trial of the 350-mm2 versus the 500-mm2 Baerveldt implant: longer term results: is bigger better? Ophthalmology. (1999). Dec;, 106(12), 2312-8.

[81] Ishida, K, Netland, P. A, Costa, V. P, Shiroma, L, Khan, B, & Ahmed, I. I. Comparison of polypropylene and silicone Ahmed Glaucoma Valves. Ophthalmology. (2006). Aug;, 113(8), 1320-6.

[82] Brasil, M. V, Rockwood, E. J, & Smith, S. D. Comparison of silicone and polypropylene Ahmed Glaucoma Valve implants. J Glaucoma. (2007). Jan;, 16(1), 36-41.

[83] Bai, Y. J, Li, Y. Q, Chai, F, Yang, X. J, Zhang, Y. C, Wei, Y. T, Huang, J. J, Ge, J, & Zhuo, Y. H. Comparison of FP-7 and S-2 Ahmed glaucoma valve implantation in re-

fractory glaucoma patients for short-term follow-up. Chin Med J (Engl). (2011). Apr;, 124(8), 1128-33.

[84] Khan, A. O, & Al-mobarak, F. Comparison of polypropylene and silicone Ahmed valve survival 2 years following implantation in the first 2 years of life.Br J Ophthalmol. (2009). Jun;, 93(6), 791-4.

[85] Hinkle, D. M, Zurakowski, D, & Ayyala, R. S. A comparison of the polypropylene plate Ahmed glaucoma valve to the silicone plate Ahmed glaucoma flexible valve. Eur J Ophthalmol. (2007). Sep-Oct;, 17(5), 696-701.

[86] Mahdy, R. A. Adjunctive use of bevacizumab versus mitomycin C with Ahmed valve implantation in treatment of pediatric glaucoma.J Glaucoma. (2011). Sep;, 20(7), 458-63.

[87] Alvarado, J. A, Hollander, D. A, Juster, R. P, & Lee, L. C. Ahmed valve implantation with adjunctive mitomycin C and 5-fluorouracil: long-term outcomes. Am J Ophthalmol. (2008). Aug;, 146(2), 276-284.

[88] Costa, V. P, Azuara-blanco, A, Netland, P. A, Lesk, M. R, & Arcieri, E. S. Efficacy and safety of adjunctive mitomycin C during Ahmed Glaucoma Valve implantation: a prospective randomized clinical trial. Ophthalmology. (2004). Jun;, 111(6), 1071-6.

[89] Kurnaz, E, Kubaloglu, A, Yilmaz, Y, Koytak, A, & Ozertürk, Y. The effect of adjunctive Mitomycin C in Ahmed glaucoma valve implantation. Eur J Ophthalmol. (2005). Jan-Feb;, 15(1), 27-31.

[90] Perkins, T. W, Gangnon, R, Ladd, W, Kaufman, P. L, & Libby, C. M. Molteno implant with mitomycin C: intermediate-term results. J Glaucoma. (1998). Apr;, 7(2), 86-92.

[91] Cantor, L, Burgoyne, J, Sanders, S, Bhavnani, V, Hoop, J, & Brizendine, E. The effect of mitomycin C on Molteno implant surgery: a 1-year randomized, masked, prospective study. J Glaucoma. (1998). Aug;, 7(4), 240-6.

[92] Costa, V. P. Surgical management. Combined cataract extraction and glaucoma drainage implant surgery. Glaucoma Saunders. (2009). , 2, 367.

[93] Seibold, L. K, Rorrer, R. A, & Kahook, M. Y. MRI of the Ex-PRESS stainless steel glaucoma drainage device. Br J Ophthalmol. (2011). Feb;, 95(2), 251-4.

[94] Geffen, N, Trope, G. E, Alasbali, T, Salonen, D, Crowley, A. P, & Buys, Y. M. Is the Ex-PRESS glaucoma shunt magnetic resonance imaging safe? J Glaucoma. (2010). Feb;, 19(2), 116-8.

[95] De Feo, F, Roccatagliata, L, Bonzano, L, Castelletti, L, Mancardi, G, & Traverso, C. E. Magnetic resonance imaging in patients implanted with Ex-PRESS stainless steel glaucoma drainage micro device. Am J Ophthalmol. (2009). May;, 147(5), 907-11.

[96] Bagnis, A, Papadia, M, Scotto, R, & Traverso, C. E. Obstruction of the Ex-PRESS miniature glaucoma device: Nd: YAG laser as a therapeutic option. J Glaucoma. (2011). Apr-May;20(4):271

[97] Dahan, E. Ben Simon GJ, Lafuma. A Comparison of trabeculectomy and Ex-PRESS Implantation in fellow eyes of the same patient: a prospective, randomised study. Eye (Lond). (2012). Feb 17.

[98] Marzette, L, & Herndon, L. W. Comparison of the Ex-PRESS™ mini glaucoma shunt with standard trabeculectomy in the surgical treatment of glaucoma. Ophthalmic Surg Lasers Imaging. (2011). Nov-Dec;, 42(6), 453-9.

[99] De Jong, L, Lafuma, A, Aguadé, A. S, & Berdeaux, G. Five-year extension of a clinical trial comparing the EX-PRESS glaucoma filtration device and trabeculectomy in primary open-angle glaucoma. Clin Ophthalmol. (2011). , 5, 527-33.

[100] Good, T. J, & Kahook, M. Y. Assessment of bleb morphologic features and postoperative outcomes after Ex-PRESS drainage device implantation versus trabeculectomy. Am J Ophthalmol. (2011). Mar;, 151(3), 507-13.

[101] De Jong, L. A. The Ex-PRESS glaucoma shunt versus trabeculectomy in open-angle glaucoma: a prospective randomized Study. Adv Ther. (2009). Mar;, 26(3), 336-45.

[102] Maris PJ JrIshida K, Netland PA. Comparison of trabeculectomy with Ex-PRESS miniature glaucoma device implanted under scleral flap.J Glaucoma. (2007). Jan;, 16(1), 14-9.

[103] Kanner, E. M, & Netland, P. A. Sarkisian SR Jr, Du H. Ex-PRESS miniature glaucoma device implanted under a scleral flap alone or combined with phacoemulsification cataract surgery..J Glaucoma (2009). Aug;, 18(6), 488-91.

[104] Lewis, R. A, Von Wolff, K, Tetz, M, Koerber, N, Kearney, J. R, Shingleton, B. J, & Samuelson, T. W. Canaloplasty: Three-year results of circumferential viscodilation and tensioning of Schlemm canal using a microcatheter to treat open-angle glaucoma. J Cataract Refract Surg. (2011). Apr;, 37(4), 682-90.

[105] Bull, H, Von Wolff, K, Körber, N, & Tetz, M. Three-year canaloplasty outcomes for the treatment of open-angle glaucoma: European study results. Graefes Arch Clin Exp Ophthalmol. (2011). Oct;, 249(10), 1537-45.

[106] Ayyala, R. S, Chaudhry, A. L, Okogbaa, C. B, & Zurakowski, D. Comparison of surgical outcomes between canaloplasty and trabeculectomy at 12 months' follow-up. Ophthalmology. (2011). Dec;, 118(12), 2427-33.

[107] Melamed, S. Ben Simon GJ, Goldenfeld M, Simon G. Efficacy and safety of gold micro shunt implantation to the supraciliary space in patients with glaucoma: a pilot study. Arch Ophthalmol. (2009). Mar;, 127(3), 264-9.

[108] Figus, M, Lazzeri, S, Fogagnolo, P, Iester, M, Martinelli, P, & Nardi, . . Supraciliary shunt in refractory glaucoma. Br J Ophthalmol. 2011 Nov;95(11):1537-41

[109] Samuelson, T. W, Katz, L. J, Wells, J. M, Duh, Y. J, & Giamporcaro, J. E. US iStent Study Group. Randomized evaluation of the trabecular micro-bypass stent with phacoemulsification in patients with glaucoma and cataract. Ophthalmology. (2011). Mar;, 118(3), 459-67.

[110] Craven, E. R, Katz, L. J, & Wells, J. M. Giamporcaro JE; iStent Study Group. Cataract surgery with trabecular micro-bypass stent implantation in patients with mild-to-moderate open-angle glaucoma and cataract: Two-year follow-up.J Cataract Refract Surg. (2012). Aug;, 38(8), 1339-45.

[111] Ting, J. L, & Damji, K. F. Stiles MC; Trabectome Study Group. Ab interno trabeculectomy: outcomes in exfoliation versus primary open-angle glaucoma. J Cataract Refract Surg. (2012). Feb;, 38(2), 315-23.

[112] Dietlein, T. S, Jordan, J. F, Schild, A, Konen, W, Jünemann, A, Lüke, C, & Krieglstein, G. K. Combined cataract-glaucoma surgery using the intracanalicular Eyepass glaucoma implant: first clinical results of a prospective pilot study. J Cataract Refract Surg. (2008). Feb;, 34(2), 247-52.

[113] Parul Ichhpujani and Marlene RMoster. Novel Glaucoma Surgical Devices. In: Shimon Rumelt (ed). Glaucoma- Basic and clinical concepts. Rijeka: InTech; (2011). , 438.

[114] Lanchulev, S, Ahmed, I, Hoeh, H, et al. Minimally invasive suprachoroidal device (Cypass) in open glaucoma. AAO (2010). poster.

[115] Craven, E. R. Khatana A Hoeh H et al. Minimally invasive ab interno suprachoroidal micro-stent for the IOP reduction in combination with phaco cataract surgery. AAO (2011). poster

[116] Lindfield, D, Ritchie, R. W, & Griffiths, M. F. Phaco-ECP': combined endoscopic cyclophotocoagulation and cataract surgery to augment medical control of glaucoma.BMJ Open. (2012). May 30;2(3). pii: e000578. doi:bmjopen-Print 2012., 2011-000578.

[117] Lima, F. E, Magacho, L, & Carvalho, D. M. Susanna R Jr, Avila MP. A prospective, comparative study between endoscopic cyclophotocoagulation and the Ahmed drainage implant in refractory glaucoma. J Glaucoma. (2004). Jun;, 13(3), 233-7.

Permissions

The contributors of this book come from diverse backgrounds, making this book a truly international effort. This book will bring forth new frontiers with its revolutionizing research information and detailed analysis of the nascent developments around the world.

We would like to thank Shimon Rumelt, for lending his expertise to make the book truly unique. He has played a crucial role in the development of this book. Without his invaluable contribution this book wouldn't have been possible. He has made vital efforts to compile up to date information on the varied aspects of this subject to make this book a valuable addition to the collection of many professionals and students.

This book was conceptualized with the vision of imparting up-to-date information and advanced data in this field. To ensure the same, a matchless editorial board was set up. Every individual on the board went through rigorous rounds of assessment to prove their worth. After which they invested a large part of their time researching and compiling the most relevant data for our readers. Conferences and sessions were held from time to time between the editorial board and the contributing authors to present the data in the most comprehensible form. The editorial team has worked tirelessly to provide valuable and valid information to help people across the globe.

Every chapter published in this book has been scrutinized by our experts. Their significance has been extensively debated. The topics covered herein carry significant findings which will fuel the growth of the discipline. They may even be implemented as practical applications or may be referred to as a beginning point for another development. Chapters in this book were first published by InTech; hereby published with permission under the Creative Commons Attribution License or equivalent.

The editorial board has been involved in producing this book since its inception. They have spent rigorous hours researching and exploring the diverse topics which have resulted in the successful publishing of this book. They have passed on their knowledge of decades through this book. To expedite this challenging task, the publisher supported the team at every step. A small team of assistant editors was also appointed to further simplify the editing procedure and attain best results for the readers.

Our editorial team has been hand-picked from every corner of the world. Their multi-ethnicity adds dynamic inputs to the discussions which result in innovative outcomes. These outcomes are then further discussed with the researchers and contributors who give their valuable feedback and opinion regarding the same. The feedback is then collaborated with the researches and they are edited in a comprehensive manner to aid the understanding of the subject.

Apart from the editorial board, the designing team has also invested a significant amount of their time in understanding the subject and creating the most relevant covers. They scrutinized every image to scout for the most suitable representation of the subject and create an appropriate cover for the book.

The publishing team has been involved in this book since its early stages. They were actively engaged in every process, be it collecting the data, connecting with the contributors or procuring relevant information. The team has been an ardent support to the editorial, designing and production team. Their endless efforts to recruit the best for this project, has resulted in the accomplishment of this book. They are a veteran in the field of academics and their pool of knowledge is as vast as their experience in printing. Their expertise and guidance has proved useful at every step. Their uncompromising quality standards have made this book an exceptional effort. Their encouragement from time to time has been an inspiration for everyone.

The publisher and the editorial board hope that this book will prove to be a valuable piece of knowledge for researchers, students, practitioners and scholars across the globe.

List of Contributors

Shimon Rumelt
Department of Ophthalmology, Western Galilee, Nahariya Medical Center, Nahariya, Israel

Cynthia Esponda-Lammoglia, Rafael Castaneda-Díez, Gerardo García-Aguirre, Oscar Albis-Donado and Jesús Jiménez-Román
Asociación para Evitar la Ceguera en México, Mexico City, Mexico

Gema Bolivar and Javier Paz Moreno-Arrones
Department of Glaucoma, Hospital Universitario Príncipe de Asturias, Alcalá de Henares, Spain

Miguel A. Teus
Department of Ophthalmology, Hospital Universitario Príncipe de Asturias, University of Alcalá, Alcalá de Henares, Spain

Marek Rękas and Karolina Krix-Jachym
Ophthalmology Department, Military Institute of Medicine, Warsaw, Poland

He-Zheng Zhou, Qian Ye, Jian-Guo Wu, Wen-Shan Jiang, Feng Chang, Yan-Ping Song, Qing Ding and Wen-Qiang Zhang
Department of Ophthalmology, Wuhan General Hospital, Guangzhou Military Command, Wuhan, China

Kin Chiu, Kwok-Fai So and Raymond Chuen-Chung Chang
Laboratory of Neurodegenerative Diseases, Department of Anatomy, LKS Faculty of Medicine, China
Research Centre of Heart, Brain, Hormone and Healthy Aging, LKS Faculty of Medicine, China
State Key Laboratory of Brain and Cognitive Sciences, The University of Hong Kong, Pokfulam, Hong Kong SAR, China

Daljit Singh
Guru Nanak Dev University, Amritsar, India

Vassilis Kozobolis, Aristeidis Konstantinidis and Georgios Labiris
Eye department, University Hospital of Alexandroupolis, Alexandroupolis, Greece

Printed in the USA
CPSIA information can be obtained
at www.ICGtesting.com
JSHW011418221024
72173JS00004B/572